W9-CLA-041

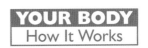

YOUR BODY
How It Works

The Nervous
System

YOUR BODY How It Works

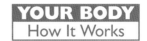

The Nervous System

F. Fay Evans-Martin, Ph.D.

Introduction by
Denton A. Cooley, M.D.
President and Surgeon-in-Chief
of the Texas Heart Institute
Clinical Professor of Surgery at the
University of Texas Medical School, Houston, Texas

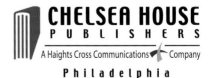

CHELSEA HOUSE
P U B L I S H E R S
A Haights Cross Communications Company
Philadelphia

To Shawn and Eric with love, to Mama and Daddy in grateful memory, and to my Creator with praise.

CHELSEA HOUSE PUBLISHERS
VP, New Product Development Sally Cheney
Director of Production Kim Shinners
Creative Manager Takeshi Takahashi
Manufacturing Manager Diann Grasse

Staff for THE NERVOUS SYSTEM
Executive Editor Tara Koellhoffer
Associate Editor Beth Reger
Editorial Assistant Kuorkor Dzani
Production Editor Noelle Nardone
Photo Editor Sarah Bloom
Series & Cover Designer Terry Mallon
Layout 21st Century Publishing and Communications, Inc.

First Printing

1 3 5 7 9 8 6 4 2

Library of Congress Cataloging-in-Publication Data

Evans-Martin, F. Fay.
   The nervous system / F. Fay Evans-Martin.
      p. cm.—(Your body, how it works)
Includes bibliographical references.
   ISBN 0-7910-7628-8
   1. Nervous system. I. Title. II. Series.
QP355.2.E94 2005
612.8—dc22

                                        2004021579

All links and web addresses were checked and verified to be correct at the time of publication. Because of the dynamic nature of the web, some addresses and links may have changed since publication and may no longer be valid.

Table of Contents

Introduction

The human body is an incredibly complex and amazing structure. At best, it is a source of strength, beauty, and wonder. We can compare the healthy body to a well-designed machine whose parts work smoothly together. We can also compare it to a symphony orchestra in which each instrument has a different part to play. When all of the musicians play together, they produce beautiful music.

From a purely physical standpoint, our bodies are made mainly of water. We are also made of many minerals, including calcium, phosphorous, potassium, sulfur, sodium, chlorine, magnesium, and iron. In order of size, the elements of the body are organized into cells, tissues, and organs. Related organs are combined into systems, including the musculoskeletal, cardiovascular, nervous, respiratory, gastrointestinal, endocrine, and reproductive systems.

Our cells and tissues are constantly wearing out and being replaced without our even knowing it. In fact, much of the time, we take the body for granted. When it is working properly, we tend to ignore it. Although the heart beats about 100,000 times per day and we breathe more than 10 million times per year, we do not normally think about these things. When something goes wrong, however, our bodies tell us through pain and other symptoms. In fact, pain is a very effective alarm system that lets us know the body needs attention. If the pain does not go away, we may need to see a doctor. Even without medical help, the body has an amazing ability to heal itself. If we cut ourselves, the blood clotting system works to seal the cut right away, and the immune defense system sends out special blood cells that are programmed to heal the area.

During the past 50 years, doctors have gained the ability to repair or replace almost every part of the body. In my own field of cardiovascular surgery, we are able to open the heart and repair its valves, arteries, chambers, and connections. In many cases, these repairs can be done through a tiny "keyhole" incision that speeds up patient recovery and leaves hardly any scar. If the entire heart is diseased, we can replace it altogether, either with a donor heart or with a mechanical device. In the future, the use of mechanical hearts will probably be common in patients who would otherwise die of heart disease.

Until the mid-twentieth century, infections and contagious diseases related to viruses and bacteria were the most common causes of death. Even a simple scratch could become infected and lead to death from "blood poisoning." After penicillin and other antibiotics became available in the 1930s and '40s, doctors were able to treat blood poisoning, tuberculosis, pneumonia, and many other bacterial diseases. Also, the introduction of modern vaccines allowed us to prevent childhood illnesses, smallpox, polio, flu, and other contagions that used to kill or cripple thousands.

Today, plagues such as the "Spanish flu" epidemic of 1918–19, which killed 20 to 40 million people worldwide, are unknown except in history books. Now that these diseases can be avoided, people are living long enough to have long-term (chronic) conditions such as cancer, heart failure, diabetes, and arthritis. Because chronic diseases tend to involve many organ systems or even the whole body, they cannot always be cured with surgery. These days, researchers are doing a lot of work at the cellular level, trying to find the underlying causes of chronic illnesses. Scientists recently finished mapping the human genome, which is a set of coded "instructions" programmed into our cells. Each cell contains 3 billion "letters" of this code. By showing how the body is made, the human genome will help researchers prevent and treat disease at its source, within the cells themselves.

The body's long-term health depends on many factors, called risk factors. Some risk factors, including our age, sex, and family history of certain diseases, are beyond our control. Other important risk factors include our lifestyle, behavior, and environment. Our modern lifestyle offers many advantages but is not always good for our bodies. In western Europe and the United States, we tend to be stressed, overweight, and out of shape. Many of us have unhealthy habits such as smoking cigarettes, abusing alcohol, or using drugs. Our air, water, and food often contain hazardous chemicals and industrial waste products. Fortunately, we can do something about most of these risk factors. At any age, the most important things we can do for our bodies are to eat right, exercise regularly, get enough sleep, and refuse to smoke, overuse alcohol, or use addictive drugs. We can also help clean up our environment. These simple steps will lower our chances of getting cancer, heart disease, or other serious disorders.

These days, thanks to the Internet and other forms of media coverage, people are more aware of health-related matters. The average person knows more about the human body than ever before. Patients want to understand their medical conditions and treatment options. They want to play a more active role, along with their doctors, in making medical decisions and in taking care of their own health.

I encourage you to learn as much as you can about your body and to treat your body well. These things may not seem too important to you now, while you are young, but the habits and behaviors that you practice today will affect your physical well-being for the rest of your life. The present book series, YOUR BODY: HOW IT WORKS, is an excellent introduction to human biology and anatomy. I hope that it will awaken within you a lifelong interest in these subjects.

Denton A. Cooley, M.D.
President and Surgeon-in-Chief
of the Texas Heart Institute
Clinical Professor of Surgery at the
University of Texas Medical School, Houston, Texas

1

Our Amazing Nervous System

INTRODUCTION

Joshua poked at the embers of his campfire as he stared at the twinkling stars in the evening sky. The taste of his dinner was still on his tongue. Wildflowers filled the air with perfume, and Joshua remembered noticing their beauty as he passed them during the day. A nearby stream trickled over the rocks, an occasional call came from a night creature, and rustling leaves revealed the presence of forest animals.

Joshua nestled into his sleeping bag and soon fell asleep, dreaming of the natural wonders he had experienced that day. While he slept, Joshua's nervous system—another natural wonder—was actively at work.

Protected within bony encasings (the skull and spinal column), the brain and spinal cord are the central core of the nervous system. A network of nerves branches out from them and acts as a fiber highway system for information coming in from the environment and going out to the muscles, glands, and body organs. Virtually every cell in the body is influenced by the nervous system in some way. In turn, the nervous system is heavily affected by hormones and other chemicals produced by cells in the body. Some of the nervous system's many jobs include regulating your breathing, heartbeat, and body temperature, controlling your movements, and even helping you digest your meals. Joshua's amazing nervous system had taken all the information his senses had collected during the day; interpreted it as beautiful sights, sounds, and aromas; and stored it for him to remember and enjoy. Every movement of his active day on the mountain trails had been under the control of this natural wonder we know as the nervous system.

NEURON THEORY

Beginning with the ancient Greek philosophers, there have been centuries of debate over the brain and its functions. It was not until the end of the 19th century that the structure and function of the nervous system began to become clear. Because nervous tissue is so soft, fragile, and complex, it was very difficult to study. Although scientists had observed and drawn nerve cells, they could not yet view all of the nerves' connections under a microscope.

In 1838, German botanist Matthias Jakob Schleiden came up with a theory that all plants are made up of individual units called cells. The next year, German physiologist Theodor Schwann introduced the theory that all animals are also made up of cells. Together, Schleiden's and Schwann's statements formed the basis of **cell theory**, which states that the cell is the basic unit that makes up the structures of all living organisms. Although cell theory quickly became popular, most scientists of the 19th century believed that the nervous system was a continuous network of fibers, or reticulum, which meant it was an exception to cell theory. This concept about the makeup of the nervous system became known as **reticular theory**.

A breakthrough came in 1873. That year, Italian scientist Camillo Golgi reported his discovery of a special stain that made **neurons** (nerve cells) and their connections easier to study under a microscope. Since his technique was not yet refined enough to see the connections between individual neurons, Golgi continued to adhere to reticular theory. He believed the nervous system was a vast network of cytoplasm with many **nuclei**.

In 1886, Swiss anatomist Wilhelm His suggested that the neuron and its connections might, in fact, be an independent unit within the nervous system. Another Swiss scientist, August Forel, proposed a similar theory a few months later. Using Golgi's staining technique and improving upon it, Spanish scientist Santiago Ramón y Cajal showed in 1888 that the neuron and its connections were indeed an individual unit within the nervous system. In a paper published in 1891, German anatomist Wilhelm Waldeyer coined the term *neurone* and introduced the neuron doctrine. Known today as **neuron theory**, Waldeyer's concept extended cell theory to nervous tissue. However, it was not until after the invention of the electron microscope in the early 1930s that definitive evidence became available to show that neurons could communicate between themselves.

Golgi and Cajal were awarded a shared Nobel Prize in Physiology or Medicine in 1906 for their scientific studies of the nervous system. At the ceremony, each man gave a speech. Golgi's speech stayed true to the reticular theory of nervous system structure. Cajal, on the other hand, spoke in enthusiastic support of neuron theory and gave evidence to contradict reticular theory. Since then, scientific studies have continued to support the neuron theory and have revealed more details that show how amazingly complex the nervous system really is. Although many questions remain to be answered, it is now clear that the nervous system is, in fact, made up of individual cells, just like the rest of the body.

THE CELLS OF THE NERVOUS SYSTEM
Neurons

The basic signaling unit of the nervous system is the neuron. Neurons are found in the brain, spinal cord, and sensory organs. Scientists estimate conservatively that there are more than 100 billion neurons in the brain and as many as 1 billion neurons in the spinal cord. Neurons come in many shapes and sizes and perform many different functions (Figures 1.1 and 1.2). Types of neurons include **unipolar neurons, bipolar neurons, pseudounipolar neurons**, and **multipolar neurons**.

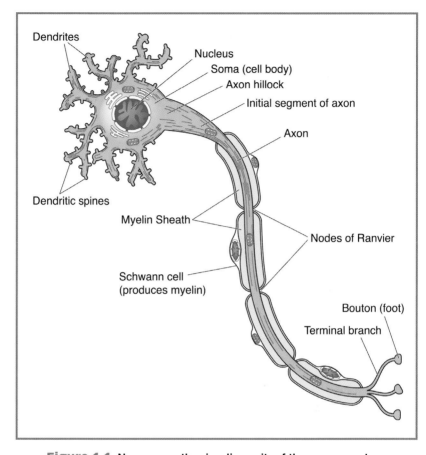

Dendrites

Nucleus

Soma (cell body)

Axon hillock

Initial segment of axon

Axon

Dendritic spines

Myelin Sheath

Nodes of Ranvier

Schwann cell
(produces myelin)

Bouton (foot)

Terminal branch

Figure 1.1 Neurons are the signaling units of the nervous system. A typical neuron is illustrated here. Neurotransmitters arrive at the dendrites, where they bind to receptors and cause tiny electrical currents that sum together at the axon hillock to generate the first of a series of action potentials that travel down the axon toward the next neuron. The myelin sheath, composed of Schwann cell processes, insulates the axon and helps the electrical impulses travel faster.

Like other cells, neurons have an outer plasma (cell) membrane that encloses the watery **cytoplasm** in which the cell **nucleus** and a variety of **organelles** are found. The nucleus is the control center of the cell. It directs the activities of the organelles, which are responsible for all of the cell's functions.

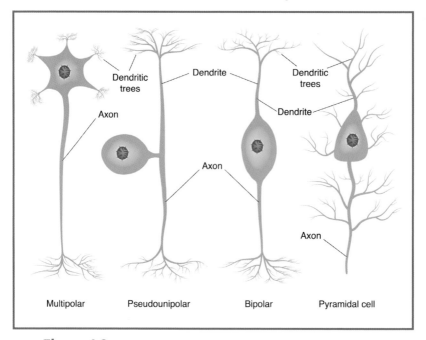

Figure 1.2 There are three basic ways in which the processes of neurons leave the cell body. Unipolar neurons (not shown) have only one process, an axon, that has multiple terminal processes. Bipolar neurons have two processes, an axon and a dendrite, that arise from opposite ends of the cell body. The pseudounipolar neuron, a type of bipolar neuron, has one fused process that branches near the soma into an axon and a dendrite. Multipolar neurons, of which the pyramidal cell is one example, have multiple dendritic trees and usually one axon.

Unlike most other cells, neurons do not divide to reproduce themselves. Also unlike most other cells, neurons are able to transmit an electrochemical signal.

Most cells in the body have geometric shapes—they are squarish, cubical, or spherical. Neurons, on the other hand, are irregular in shape and have a number of extensions (sometimes called "processes") coming off them. This makes them look something like a many-legged spider. The neuron's extensions send and receive information to and from other neurons.

Usually, each neuron has only one **axon**, an extension that carries messages away from the cell. Although a neuron's body is usually just 5 to 100 micrometers in diameter, axons can range in length from 1 millimeter to as long as 1 meter. Sometimes axons branch into one or more collateral axons. Each axon may have several small branches at the end; these are called axon terminals.

On the opposite side of the neuron cell body are shorter extensions called **dendrites** that branch like trees. In fact, their arrangement is referred to as the "dendritic tree." Dendrites receive messages from other neurons. A single neuron can have anywhere from 1 to 20 dendrites, each of which can branch many times.

Dendritic spines are short, knobby structures that appear on the dendrites. There may be thousands of dendritic spines on just one neuron. This greatly increases the surface area that the dendritic tree has available for receiving signals from other neurons. To relay messages, axons from different neurons contact the dendrites, the dendritic spines, and the cell body. Together, these structures receive information from as many as 10,000 other neurons. Axons can also end on a muscle, another axon, a tiny blood vessel, or in the **extracellular fluid** (the watery space that surrounds cells). Many **neurotransmitters** are synthesized and stored in the axon terminals. Some are synthesized in the cell body and transported down the axon to the terminals. When released, neurotransmitters carry chemical messages between neurons and to muscle fibers, which they cause to contract. They also carry messages to organs and glands that affect the function of all the body systems. Dendrites can also connect to another dendrite to communicate with it.

Glia

Glia are special cells that play a supportive role in the nervous system. They outnumber neurons by about 10 to 1 in the brain, where they make up half or more of the brain's volume. The number of glia in other parts of the nervous system has not yet been determined. Like neurons, glia have many extensions coming off their cell bodies. Unlike neurons, however, glia probably do not send out electrochemical signals. Also unlike neurons, glia are replaced constantly throughout a person's life.

Astrocytes are one type of glia. They surround neurons and, at the same time, contact blood vessels. Astrocytes provide nutritional support to neurons and help keep most substances other than oxygen, carbon dioxide, glucose, and essential amino acids from entering the brain from the bloodstream. Astrocytes give structural support to hold neurons in place and also scavenge dead cells after an injury to the brain. In addition, astrocytes contribute to the formation of the **blood-brain barrier**, which protects the brain from toxins, peripheral neurotransmitters, and other substances that would interfere with the brain's functioning.

Processes from astrocytes called "end feet" adhere to the blood vessels of the brain and secrete chemical signals that induce (cause) the formation of tight junctions between the endothelial cells which line the blood vessels. As a result, substances from the extracellular fluid cannot move easily into these cells. The small pores called fenestrations, and some of the transport mechanisms that are present in peripheral blood vessels are also absent.

Most large molecules cannot cross this blood-brain barrier. Small fat-soluble molecules and uncharged particles

THE BRAIN'S CLEANUP CREW

Small cells called **microglia** migrate from the blood into the brain. They act as the cleanup crew when nerve cells die. They also produce chemicals called growth factors that help damaged neurons to heal. When you view a damaged area of the brain under a microscope, you can see glial cells clustered in the places where dead cells were removed.

such as carbon dioxide and oxygen, however, diffuse easily across this barrier. Glucose and essential amino acids are transported across by special transporter proteins. Toxins that can diffuse across the blood-brain barrier include nerve gases, alcohol, and nicotine.

Other glial cells include **oligodendrocytes** and **Schwann cells**. These cells provide electrical insulation for axons. They have fewer extensions than astrocytes do. Like astrocytes, they also help bring nutritional support to neurons. Schwann cells help repair damaged nerves outside the brain and spinal cord.

Ependymal cells are glial cells that line the **ventricles**, or fluid-filled cavities of the brain. Unlike other glial cells, they do not have processes coming off the cell body. They secrete cerebrospinal fluid, the liquid that fills the ventricles and the spinal canal. The spinal canal runs through the center of the spinal cord and is continuous with the **ventricular system** of the brain. Cerebrospinal fluid acts as a shock-absorbing cushion to protect the brain from blows to the head. In effect, this fluid makes the brain float inside the skull. The cerebrospinal fluid also removes waste products from the brain.

THE NERVE SIGNAL

The plasma membrane of the neuron is made up of a double layer, or bilayer, of lipids, or fatty molecules, called the phospholipid bilayer. Since oil (or fat) and water "don't mix," this bilayer forms a barrier between the water outside the cell and the water inside the cell. It also keeps substances that are dissolved in water—for example, charged atoms called ions—from crossing the cell membrane. Very few substances can cross this lipid bilayer easily.

Wedged between the fatty molecules of the plasma membrane are many proteins. Some of these proteins have pores, or channels, that let certain ions enter the cell. Some channels are open all the time to let particular ions move back and forth. These channels are said to be ungated. Other channels stay closed unless they get a message, such as an electrical signal, that causes them to open. These are referred to as gated channels.

Protein molecules, which are kept inside the cell, have a negative charge. As a result, they give the entire cell a negative charge as compared to the extracellular fluid. The concentration of certain ions differs between the inside of the neuron, or intracellular space, and the extracellular fluid. The inside of the cell has more potassium (K+) ions, whereas the outside of the cell has more sodium (Na$^+$) and chloride (Cl$^-$) ions. A special protein in the plasma membrane helps control how much sodium and potassium is in the cell by pumping potassium ions in and sodium ions out (Figure 1.3).

The inside of the plasma membrane is about 70 millivolts more negative than the outside of the cell membrane. This electrical charge is called the resting potential of the membrane. The interior of the cell membrane is said to be "polarized." When an electrical charge or a particular chemical causes channels for sodium ions to open, sodium ions pour into the cell. This makes the inside of the cell membrane more positive, or "depolarized." If enough sodium ions enter the cell to bring down the electrical potential by about 20 millivolts—to what is called the threshold potential—there is a sudden, dramatic change in the voltage difference across the membrane. At this point, when voltage on the inside of the membrane is then 50 millivolts more *negative* than that on the outside, the interior voltage makes a sudden reversal, which continues until the voltage inside the membrane is 30 millivolts more *positive* than that outside the membrane.

This sudden reversal in voltage is called an **action potential**. It lasts for about one millisecond. The change in voltage lets potassium ions leave the cell more freely, which causes a loss of positive charge and leads to a sudden reversal of the voltage inside the membrane back to a level that is slightly more negative than the resting potential. The drop in voltage below that of the resting potential is called **hyperpolarization**.

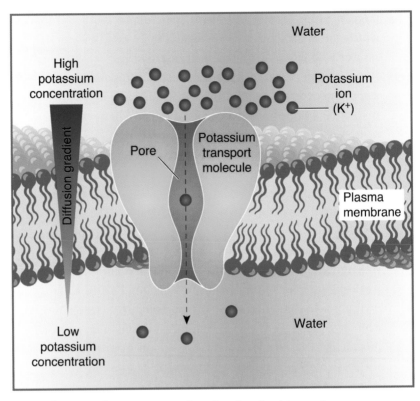

Figure 1.3 Few ions and molecules, besides water, oxygen, and carbon dioxide, can get through the lipid bilayer of the cell membrane. Because of this, other substances that are needed for cell function require the help of special proteins that span the lipid bilayer to help them pass through. Shown here is the transporter for the positively charged potassium ion, which responds to depolarization by allowing potassium ions to leave the cell, thereby restoring the polarization of the interior of the cell membrane.

After the action potential has finished firing, the voltage inside the membrane slowly returns to the resting potential.

THE SYNAPSE

How does a nerve signal travel from one neuron to another? Between the tip of each axon terminal and the point on the target neuron (usually a dendritic spine or the cell body) to which the axon sends a nerve signal, there is a tiny gap. It measures about 10 to 20 nanometers across, and is called the synaptic cleft. The term **synapse** refers to the **synaptic cleft** and the areas on the two neurons that are involved in the transmission and reception of a chemical signal. The presynaptic neuron is the one that sends the message. It releases a neurotransmitter into the synaptic cleft. Every neuron produces one or more kinds of neurotransmitters and stores them inside spherical-shaped structures in the membrane called synaptic vesicles until the neuron receives a neural signal. The synaptic vesicles then move to the presynaptic membrane, bind to it, and release their contents into the synaptic cleft. Neurotransmitters diffuse across the synaptic cleft and bind to a particular receptor, or membrane protein, found on the surface of the plasma membrane of the postsynaptic (receiving) neuron (Figure 1.4). The neurotransmitter fits into the receptor protein like a key in a lock, and causes an ion channel to open.

As sodium ions enter the postsynaptic neuron through the activated ion channels, tiny electrical currents are produced. These currents travel to the place where the cell body meets the

THE REFRACTORY PERIOD

An action potential only travels in one direction down the axon. The reason for this is that there is a **refractory period** that begins immediately after the firing of an action potential. It lasts for several milliseconds. During the first portion of this refractory period, called the absolute refractory period, the neuron cannot fire again, because sodium channels have been left inactive. As the efflux of potassium ions pushes the voltage below the threshold potential, a relative refractory period occurs. During this time, a greater depolarization than usual is needed to cause an action potential to fire.

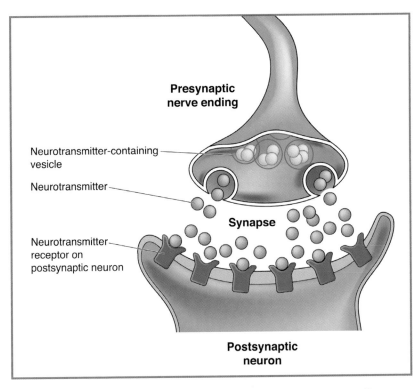

Presynaptic nerve ending

Neurotransmitter-containing vesicle

Neurotransmitter

Synapse

Neurotransmitter receptor on postsynaptic neuron

Postsynaptic neuron

Figure 1.4 The synapse is the tiny space between a nerve ending and the neuron with which it communicates. Neurotransmitters carry the nerve signal as a chemical message across the synapse from the first (presynaptic) neuron to the second (postsynaptic) neuron. They bind to receptors on the postsynaptic cell membrane.

axon, a site called the **axon hillock**. There, the tiny electrical currents join together. Each neuron receives thousands of neural signals per second from other neurons. Some of them are excitatory and open sodium channels. Others are inhibitory and open chloride or potassium channels. Depending on the number and type of tiny electrical currents generated as the neurotransmitter chemicals bind to the receptors of the postsynaptic membrane, the axon hillock gets a message to fire or not to fire an action potential. It fires an action potential only if there are enough currents to open a large enough number of voltage-gated sodium channels to make the membrane over the axon hillock reach its threshold potential.

As the action potential travels down the axon, away from the cell body, it makes the voltage of the area near the axonal membrane more positive. In turn, this opens voltage-gated ion channels. As the voltage of the adjoining intracellular membrane drops to its threshold potential, another action potential fires. This process continues until a series of action potentials travels the length of the axon.

Some axons, especially those that have to travel longer distances, are myelinated. **Myelin** is a covering of glial extensions that wrap around and around the axon of a neuron in layers. This covering forms what is called a myelin sheath. The layers of myelin provide additional electrical insulation. This extra insulation lets nerve impulses travel very fast in a myelinated axon—up to 120 meters (more than the length of a football field) per second. The extra insulation provided by the myelin sheath also helps an action potential travel much farther in a myelinated axon. In the brain and spinal cord, each oligodendrocyte may wrap its processes around segments of up to 50 axons. In the nerves outside the brain and spinal cord, Schwann cell processes wrap around one part of the axon of just one neuron. An unmyelinated axon has only the lipid bilayer of its own plasma membrane for electrical insulation.

Each myelinated segment measures about 0.1 to 0.5 micrometers in length. Between these segments are tiny unmyelinated gaps called the **nodes of Ranvier**. At these nodes, sodium ions enter through voltage-gated ion channels to propagate, or reproduce, the action potential. As a new action potential is generated at each node of Ranvier, the neural signal appears to "jump" from one node to the next.

CONNECTIONS

The nervous system is an intricate network of neurons (nerve cells) and their connections. Surrounding the neurons are glia, which play many supportive roles in the nervous system. Neurons receive and process chemical messages from other neurons and then send electrical signals down their axons to trigger the release of neurotransmitters, chemical messengers that go out to other neurons. The electrical current that travels down the neuronal axon is made up of action potentials, which are generated by the opening of voltage-gated sodium channels in the axonal membrane.

2

Development of the Nervous System

Considering that our brains help us do just about everything in our lives, it should come as no surprise that the brain itself grows at an incredibly fast rate well before we are born. The first visible signs of the developing nervous system show up during the third week after conception. At this point, the embryo consists of three layers of cells: an outer layer called the *ectoderm*, a middle layer called the *mesoderm*, and an inner layer called the *endoderm*. The ectoderm will develop into the nervous system as well as the hair, skin, and nails that cover our bodies. The mesoderm will develop into muscle, bone, and connective tissue as well as some of the internal organs, including the heart and blood vessels. From the endoderm, the digestive and respiratory tracts and additional internal organs develop.

Around day 16 of development, a thickened layer of cells, called the neural plate, appears in the midline of the **dorsal** surface of the ectodermal layer. (Since we walk upright, the term *dorsal* corresponds to the **posterior**, or backside, in human beings. The term *ventral* refers to the opposite, or **anterior**, surface—the front side of a person.)

As the neural plate develops, the cells at its edges multiply faster than the rest. This makes the plate's edges curve upward to form a neural groove in the center. By day 21 of development, the edges of the two sides of the neural plate meet and join to form the **neural tube**. This fusion begins at the place where the neck region will eventually be located. It then continues to join **rostrally** (toward the head end) and **caudally** (toward the tail end) until the whole dorsal surface of the tube is fused. Finally, the rostral and caudal ends of the neural tube close on day 24 and day 26, respectively. This process of forming the neural tube is known as primary neurulation (Figure 2.1).

The adult spinal cord can be divided into five regions, from the neck down: cervical, thoracic, lumbar, sacral, and coccygeal. The cervical, thoracic, and lumbar segments of the spinal cord develop from the neural tube. The sacral and coccygeal segments, on the other hand, develop from the caudal eminence, a cell mass located caudal to the neural tube. It appears around day 20 and grows larger, then forms a cavity before it joins the neural tube. This process, called secondary neurulation, is completed by day 42.

As the neural tube closes, cells separate from the upper edges, or crests, of the neural folds to form the neural crest. From the neural crest, parts of the **peripheral nervous system** will develop. (The peripheral nervous system includes all the nerves and neurons outside the brain and spinal cord.) Cells from the neural crest move to a position on either side of the neural tube. Sensory neurons, the **adrenal medulla**, peripheral neurons and glia of the **autonomic nervous system**, along with the two inner layers of the protective lining, or **meninges**, that cover the brain, all develop from neural crest cells. The outer layer of the meningeal covering of the brain forms from the mesoderm.

By the sixth week after conception, the nervous system has already developed to its basic form. The major structures are all recognizable by the tenth week. All brain structures are present in an immature form by the end of the first trimester (first three months). During the first three months of fetal development, the vertebral column and spinal cord grow at about the same rate. The nerves from the spinal cord exit directly through openings in the vertebral column called **intervertebral foramina**. After this point, however, the vertebral column grows faster than the spinal cord. This leaves a space called the **lumbar cistern** in the lower part of the vertebral

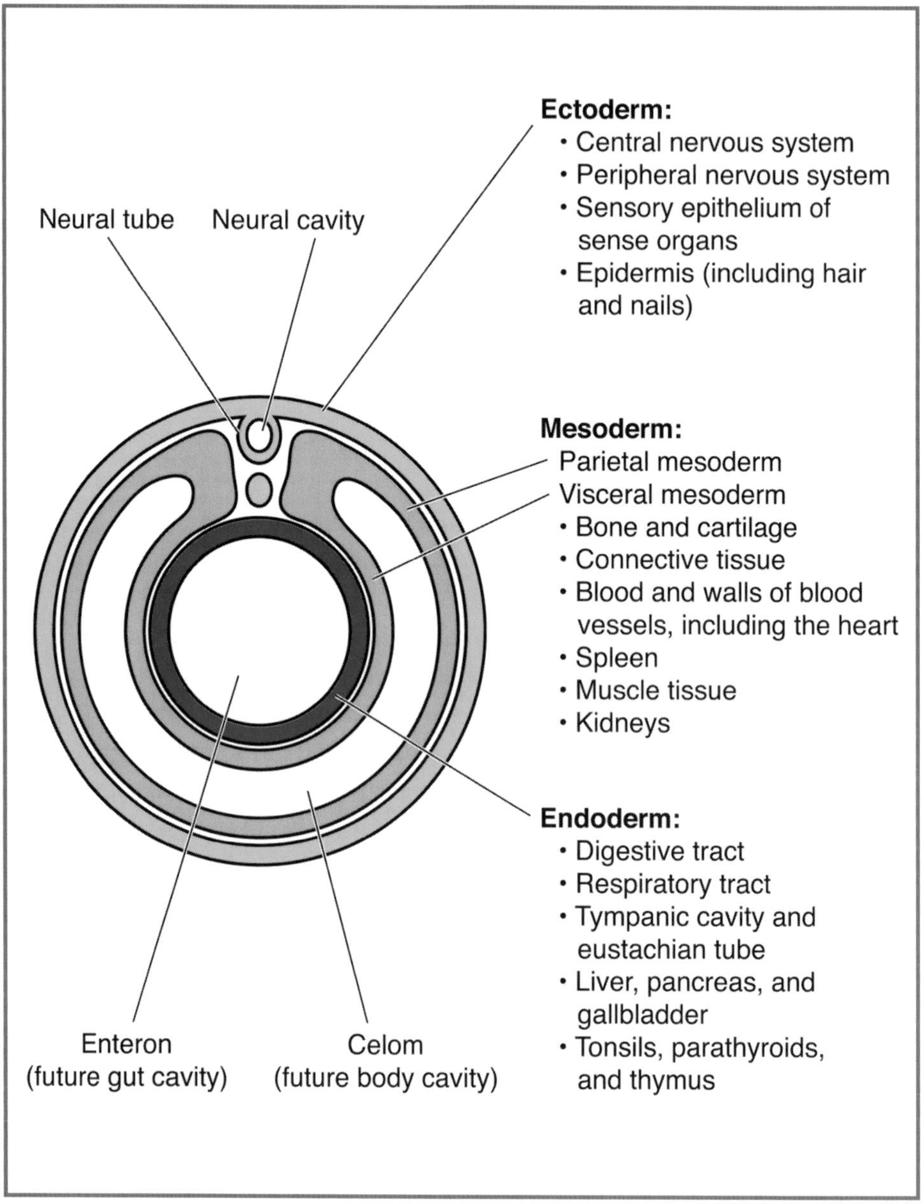

Ectoderm:
• Central nervous system
• Peripheral nervous system
• Sensory epithelium of sense organs
• Epidermis (including hair and nails)

Neural tube   Neural cavity

Mesoderm:
Parietal mesoderm
Visceral mesoderm
• Bone and cartilage
• Connective tissue
• Blood and walls of blood vessels, including the heart
• Spleen
• Muscle tissue
• Kidneys

Endoderm:
• Digestive tract
• Respiratory tract
• Tympanic cavity and eustachian tube
• Liver, pancreas, and gallbladder
• Tonsils, parathyroids, and thymus

Enteron
(future gut cavity)

Celom
(future body cavity)

Figure 2.1 This diagram shows the neural tube just after neurulation. Notice that the primary germ layers—the ectoderm, endoderm, and mesoderm—are still present. Each layer gives rise to a specific set of structures in the developing body.

canal that is not filled by the spinal cord. Spinal nerves associated with the foramina in the area of the lumbar cistern travel down from their origin in the spinal cord through the lumbar cistern before they leave through their associated foramina.

At birth, the brain weighs 400 grams (0.88 lbs) on average. By age 3, the weight of the brain has tripled, due to myelination of axons and development of neuronal processes and synaptic connections. By the time a person is 11 years old, the brain has reached its maximum weight, which can vary from 1,100 to 1,700 grams (2.4 to 3.7 lbs). The average human brain weighs about 1,400 grams (3 lbs). After age 50, people experience a

WHAT IS NEUROGENESIS?

Scientists once thought that a human infant was born with all the neurons it would ever have and that no new neurons were produced after birth. You can imagine the ripples in the scientific world in 1998 when Peter S. Eriksson, Fred H. Gage, and their colleagues announced their discovery of **neurogenesis**— the production of new neurons in the adult brain. These scientists injected bromodeoxyuridine, a thymidine analog (molecule with a similar structure) that is incorporated into newly formed DNA, into terminally ill patients and examined their brains after they died. He and his fellow researchers found neurons in the hippocampus that were stained by this molecular marker, which indicated that they had been produced after the injection. Later research has detected the migration of stem cells from the subventricular zone (SVZ) to sites in the cerebral cortex. The SVZ is a layer of cells that lies underneath the ependymal layer in the walls of the lateral ventricles. Related studies in rodents have shown that exercise, enriched environments, and learning enhance neurogenesis and that stress and inflammation reduce it. Scientists hope that neurogenesis research will eventually yield answers that will help restore or regenerate brains afflicted with neurodegenerative disease.

gradual decrease in brain weight, which may cause a slow decline in some cognitive, or thinking, functions.

DEVELOPMENTAL NEUROLOGICAL DISORDERS

Approximately 40% of all infant deaths before the first birthday happen because something goes wrong with the development of the central nervous system. A leading cause of death shortly after birth are neural tube defects. In fact, problems with neural tube development are the leading cause of infant deaths (second only to heart defects). If the neural tube does not close properly, the nervous system may not be correctly formed. This occurs in about 1 out of every 1,000 live births. Most fetuses with major nervous system malformations die before or within the first year after birth.

Spina bifida is a birth defect that results when the neural tube does not close completely at the caudal (tail) end. Depending on how severe the condition is, the overlying vertebrae and tissue may not develop, which lets the meninges and spinal cord protrude to the surface of the back. Spina bifida may also cause varying degrees of leg paralysis and problems with bladder control.

Anencephaly is a birth defect that can result when the rostral (head) end of the neural tube does not close all the way. When this happens, the cerebral hemispheres will be partially absent, and some of the overlying bone and tissue may not form as well. When a baby is born with this condition, it is usually blind, deaf, and unconscious. It may also have no ability to feel pain. Infants with anencephaly almost always die within hours—or, at most, days—after they are born.

Chromosomal abnormalities can cause problems in brain development. One example is Down's syndrome, which occurs in 1 out of 700 infants. The children of mothers who are over age 45 at the time of birth are more likely to suffer from Down's syndrome—the chances are 1 in 25 as compared to 1 in 1,550 for mothers under the age of 20. Babies born with

Down's syndrome have an extra copy of chromosome 21. Because of this, the disorder is sometimes called trisomy 21. Symptoms of Down's syndrome include mental retardation, flattened facial features, stubby hands, short stature, an open mouth, and a round head.

Fragile X syndrome is an inherited developmental disorder that results from a mutant gene on the X chromosome. Symptoms include mental retardation, an elongated face with a large jaw, enlarged testes (in males), and flared ears.

Other developmental abnormalities can result from malnutrition or from exposure to radiation, environmental toxins, drugs, and some pathogens (organisms that cause infections). Viruses (such as rubella and cytomegalovirus), bacteria (such as the spirochete bacterium that causes syphilis), and protozoans (such as *Toxoplasma*, which is found in garden dirt and cat feces) can all lead to nervous system defects. Drugs used to treat epilepsy can cause defective neural tube development. Neonatal exposure to lead or mercury can lead to neurological problems. If the mother smokes, drinks alcohol, or takes cocaine or other drugs of abuse during her pregnancy, it can also cause problems in neurological development. There is evidence that cocaine, for example, interferes with the myelination of axons in adults.

Because there is an intimate relationship between the nervous system and the structures of the skin, bone, muscles, and meninges, when someone has a defect in nervous system development, he or she usually has problems in other areas as well. Defects in facial features often accompany problems in brain development. This is particularly true in cases of fetal alcohol syndrome, which can occur if the mother drinks alcohol while she is pregnant. Children with fetal alcohol syndrome often have slit-like eyes, a thin upper lip, and a small face. They may also have behavioral and cognitive problems as well as other birth defects, such as hearing impairments, heart defects, and speech impediments.

CONNECTIONS

The nervous system starts to develop during the third week after conception. The neural plate appears first, then folds to form the neural tube. Neural crest cells separate from the neural tube as it closes to form what will become the peripheral nervous system. By the fifth week, the five major areas of the brain have developed as pouches that come off the neural tube. As the walls of the neural tube thicken and form the future brain structures, the cavity of the neural tube grows into the ventricular system of the brain. Neurons that will make up the brain structures move from the inner lining of the neural cavity to their final destinations. Ten weeks after conception, all the major brain structures are recognizable. It was once thought that at birth, a person already had all the neurons that he or she would have for a lifetime. However, recent discoveries of the formation of new neurons (neurogenesis) in the adult human brain has changed that. Myelination also continues to occur into adulthood. Synaptic changes take place throughout life as well. Problems with the closure of the neural tube or in the migration of neurons result in birth defects. Injury or exposure to toxins can also cause developmental disorders in the growing nervous system.

3

Organization of the Nervous System

The complexity of the human nervous system, particularly the brain, is such that the most sophisticated computers have been unable to emulate it. Every moment of the day, neural messages are speeding through neural pathways between the various components of the nervous system. We are unaware of most of these messages as they regulate the vital functions and rhythms of our bodies. These messages bring us information about our environment, process it, and store it for future use. They also enable us to respond to and manipulate our environment. Communication and thinking are made possible by the synchronization of many neural messages. Let's take a look at how the brain and the rest of the nervous system work together to make all of this possible.

DIVISIONS OF THE NERVOUS SYSTEM

The nervous system is divided into the central nervous system (CNS) and the peripheral nervous system (Figure 3.1). Table 3.1 shows how the central and peripheral nervous systems are organized. The central nervous system consists of the brain and spinal cord, which lie within the bones of the skull and vertebral column. The peripheral nervous system includes all the components of the nervous system that lie outside the brain and spinal cord. Axons from neurons in the brain travel down the spinal cord and out to their targets. These axons travel in bundles within fiber tracts (pathways) down the spinal cord and then travel out to their targets through the peripheral nerves. Sensory fibers from different parts of the body travel in the opposite direction through the peripheral nerves to the spinal cord and up to their targets in the brain.

Table 3.1 DIVISIONS OF THE NERVOUS SYSTEM

Central Nervous System

> ➤ Brain

> ➤ Spinal Cord

Peripheral Nervous System

> ➤ Autonomic Nervous System

> • Parasympathetic Nervous System

> • Sympathetic Nervous System

> • Enteric Nervous System

> ➤ Somatic Nervous System

> • Sensory Neurons

> • Motor Nerves

THE CENTRAL NERVOUS SYSTEM
The Brain

The Cerebrum

The major divisions of the brain are the cerebrum, diencephalon, brainstem, and cerebellum (Figure 3.2). The two

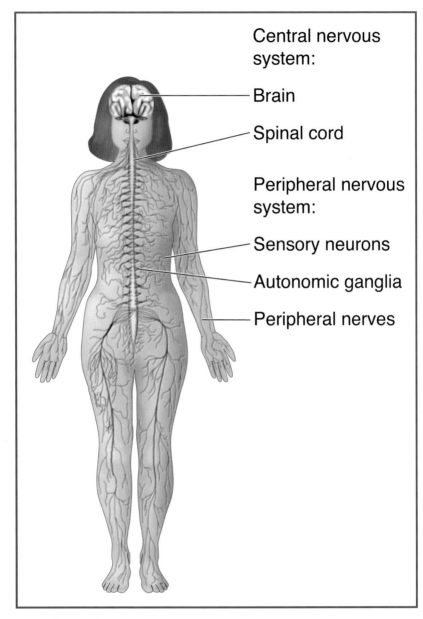

Figure 3.1 The central and peripheral nervous systems are illustrated here. The central nervous system consists of the brain and spinal cord, while the sensory and ganglionic neurons and the peripheral nerves make up the peripheral nervous system.

halves of the cerebrum, or the cerebral hemispheres, form the largest portion of the brain. They are covered by the **cerebral cortex** (*cortex* means "bark" or "rind"), a thin layer of **gray matter** that is about 3 millimeters (0.12 inches) deep. (*Gray matter* is the term used to describe the areas where the neurons are densest and the cell bodies give the brain a grayish-brown color.) It is organized into ridges (gyri) and fissures (sulci), that make it look something like a crumpled piece of paper. Underneath the cerebral cortex is a much deeper layer of fiber tracts with axons that travel to and from the cortex. This layer is called **white matter**. It has a whitish appearance, due to the myelin in the axons.

In each hemisphere, the cerebral cortex is divided into four lobes on each side by deep fissures. The first is the central sulcus, which crosses the cortex and extends horizontally

WHAT IS LATERALIZATION OF FUNCTION?

Lateralization of function, or **hemispheric dominance**, refers to the dominant role of one or the other cerebral hemisphere in a particular function. For some functions, such as fine motor control and sensory input, neither hemisphere is dominant—the hemisphere opposite to the body structure is in charge. For example, the right hemisphere sends the commands that control the movement of the left fingers and receives sensory information from the left side of the body. However, one hemisphere may be more important in controlling certain functions than the other. That hemisphere is said to be dominant for a particular function. Language is a function for which the left hemisphere is dominant for over 95% of people. Other functions for which the left hemisphere is usually dominant are calculations and recognition of details. Recognizing faces, expression and experiencing of emotions, as well as visual-spatial abilities, are functions for which the right hemisphere is dominant.

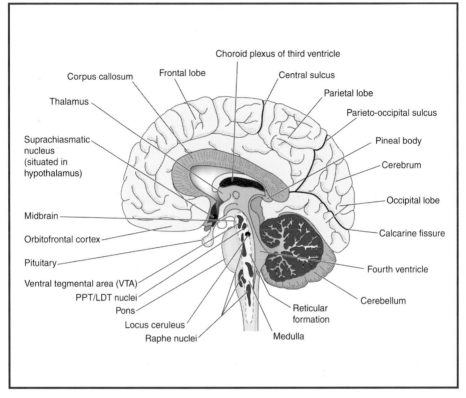

Figure 3.2 This is a midsagital view of the brain and is what you would see if the brain were cut down the the middle between the two cerebral hemispheres. The corpus callosum is the fiber bundle that connects the two hemispheres and allows them to exchange information. Most structures of the brain are paired: There is one on each side of the brain.

down to the lateral sulcus, which defines the upper limit of the **temporal lobe**. Above the temporal lobe and in front of (rostral to) the central sulcus is the **frontal lobe**. Behind (caudal to) the frontal lobe and bounded on the rear by the **parieto-occipital sulcus** (the fissure separating the occipital and parietal lobes) is the **parietal lobe**. The **occipital lobe** surrounds the posterior pole (center back) of the cerebral cortex and is bounded at the front by the parieto-occipital sulcus and an imaginary line that goes from the edge of the parieto-occipital sulcus down to the occipital notch. An imaginary line that runs from the edge of the lateral sulcus to intersect at right angles with this line marks the lower boundary of the parietal lobe.

The frontal lobe controls thinking, speech, emotion, and the production and planning of movements. The occipital lobe receives and interprets input from the eyes. The parietal lobe receives sensory messages from the skin, joints, and muscles and interprets them as pain, touch, and the position of our arms and legs in space. Auditory (hearing) and visual inputs are also integrated with these **somatosensory** messages in the parietal lobe. Primary auditory input goes to the temporal lobe, which interprets it as sound. The temporal lobe plays a role in feeling emotion, perceiving form and color, and understanding speech. The temporal lobe also houses areas to which the olfactory (sense of smell) tract projects after it crosses the ventral surface of the brain.

Six layers of neurons in the cerebral cortex send and receive messages through a large network of axons that fan out under the cortex. These axons come together into fiber tracts that descend toward the brainstem. Fibers also connect the two cerebral hemispheres and form a dense structure called the **corpus callosum**, which arches above the lateral ventricles. Table 3.2 shows the different structures of the brain and how they are organized.

Deep in the cerebral hemispheres are several important nuclei, or groups of neurons with similar functions. In the temporal lobe, the **hippocampus**, which is associated with emotion and memory, forms the medial wall and floor of the lateral ventricle. In front of the anterior tip of the hippocampus is the **amygdala**, which helps us express emotion and generate a response to stressful events. The **basal ganglia** (clusters of neurons) are important in motor function control. A group of these lies deep in the cerebrum, close to each lateral ventricle.

Table 3.2 ANATOMICAL DIVISIONS AND STRUCTURES OF THE BRAIN

DIVISION	VENTRICLE	SUBDIVISION	MAJOR STRUCTURES
Forebrain	Lateral	Telencephalon	Cerebral Cortex Basal Ganglia Amygdala Hippocampus Septal Nuclei
	Third	Diencephalon	Thalamus Hypothalamus
Brainstem:			

Midbrain	Cerebral Aqueduct	Mesencephalon	Tectum (roof):
			    Superior Collicui
			    Inferior Colliculi
			
			Cerebral Peduncles
			
			Tegmentum (floor):
			    Rostral Reticular Formation
			    Periaqueductal Gray Matter
			    Red Nucleus
			    Ventral Tegmental Area
			    Substantia Nigra
			    Locus Coeruleus Nuclei
			    PPT/LDT Nuclei
			    Cranial Nerve Nuclei III, IV, V

Hindbrain	Fourth	Metencephalon	Cerebellum
			
			Pons:
			    Reticular Formation
			    Raphe Nuclei
			    Cranial Nerve Nuclei V, VI, VII, VIII

		Myelencephalon	Medulla oblongata:
			    Reticular Formation
			    Raphe Nuclei
			    Cranial Nerve Nuclei V, VII, VIII, IX, X, XII

*   One of the CN V nuclei, the spinal trigeminal nucleus, extends into the caudal pons from the dorsal column of the spinal cord, with which it is continuous. The nucleus of Cranial Nerve XI, which exits from the medulla, is located just below the junction of the medulla with the spinal cord.

One of the basal ganglia is a C-shaped structure called the caudate nucleus. It actually forms the lateral wall and floor of the main body of the ventricle in each cerebral hemisphere.

The Diencephalon

Beneath the cerebral hemispheres and on either side of the third ventricle are paired groups of nuclei called the **thalamus** and **hypothalamus** (known together as the diencephalon). Some of the nuclei of the hypothalamus are also found in the floor of the third ventricle. All inputs from the sense organs, except those associated with smell, synapse on nuclei in the thalamus, which then relay information to the cerebral cortex. Some of the functions of the hypothalamus include control of the release of hormones from the **pituitary gland** and integration of the functions of the autonomic nervous system.

The Brainstem

Moving downward from the base of the diencephalon, the three divisions of the **brainstem** are the **midbrain, pons**, and **medulla**. Throughout the length of the brainstem, a web-like network of neurons called the **reticular formation** lies beneath the floor of the fourth ventricle. Within the reticular formation are several areas that relate to cardiovascular and respiratory control, sleep, consciousness, and alertness. Because these are such critical functions, damage to the brainstem can be lethal.

Areas of the midbrain play a role in eye movement, the perception of pain, regulation of body temperature, and the organization of simple movements. Along with the pons, the midbrain also helps control the sleep/wake cycle. Within the pons are areas that initiate dreaming and sleep, regulate our level of attention, and integrate the sensory and motor functions of the ear, eye, tongue, and facial muscles. The medulla controls limb position and head orientation, regulates breathing and heart rate, and integrates certain reflexes, such as sneezing, swallowing, and coughing.

Ten of the nuclei of the cranial nerves (*cranial* refers to the skull), which perform sensory and motor functions for the head and neck, are found in the brainstem (Table 3.3). All of the cranial nerves are considered to be part of the peripheral nervous system. However, the olfactory bulb and tract and the optic nerve are both considered to be part of the central nervous system as well.

Table 3.3 THE FUNCTIONS OF CRANIAL NERVES

CRANIAL NERVE	MAIN FUNCTIONS
I. Olfactory	Smell
II. Optic	Sight
III. Oculomotor	Eye movements, and function of the pupil and lens
IV. Trochlear	Eye movements
V. Trigeminal	Facial sensation and chewing
VI. Abducens	Eye movements
VII. Facial	Taste and facial expression
VIII. Vestibulocochlear	Hearing and equilibrium
IX. Glossopharyngeal	Taste and swallowing
X. Vagus	Speech, swallowing, and visceral sensory and motor functions
XI. Accessory	Head and shoulder movements
XII. Hypoglossal	Tongue movements

The Cerebellum

Sitting atop the fourth ventricle is the **cerebellum**—a structure that looks very much like a smaller cerebrum. Like the cerebral hemispheres, the cerebellum is made up of a thin, folded cortex, underlying fiber tracts, and groups of deep, paired nuclei. The cerebellum performs several critical functions. These include coordination of movements, maintenance of posture, and the learning of motor skills. There is also evidence that the cerebellum may be involved in higher processes, such as thinking, reasoning, memory, speech, and emotions. High levels of alcohol (which is toxic) affect the cerebellum and cause a person to stagger and to display a wide stance to keep his or her balance. Because alcohol produces these typical effects, traffic officers often require people suspected of drinking and driving to try to walk a straight line, which is very difficult to do under the influence of alcohol.

The Spinal Cord

The spinal cord makes up only about 2% of the volume of the central nervous system, but it is very important for many functions. It acts as a pathway for sensory input to the brain. Neurons located in the spinal cord send commands to muscles and internal organs. These neurons, in turn, are regulated by messages from the brain that travel down the spinal cord. In a sense, the spinal cord is the link between the brain and the body.

The medulla transitions to the spinal cord at an opening called the **foramen magnum** at the base of the skull. The spinal cord takes up two-thirds of the length of the spinal canal and measures 42 to 45 cm (16.5 to 17.7 inches) long, with a diameter of about 1 cm (0.4 inches) at its widest point. It consists of 31 segments: 8 in the cervical region, 12 in the thoracic region, 5 in the lumbar region, 5 in the sacral region, and 1 in the coccygeal region. Each segment of the spinal cord attaches to a pair of spinal nerves. Each spinal nerve has both a dorsal root made up of incoming sensory fibers and a ventral root made up of nerve fibers that go out to the muscles (Figure 3.3). The dorsal root contains fibers from a **dorsal root ganglion**, which is a cluster of neurons close to the point where the spinal nerve attaches to the spinal cord. The ventral

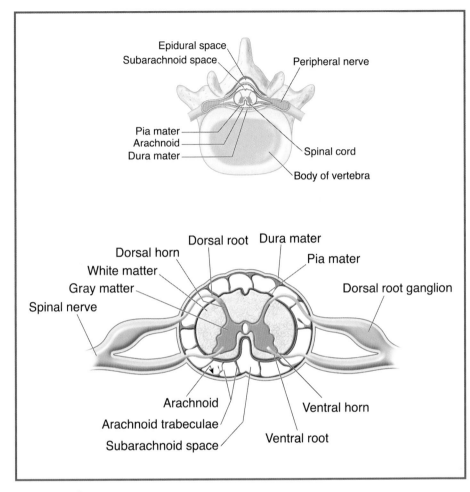

Figure 3.3 Illustrated here is a horizontal section of the spinal cord, showing the butterfly-shaped gray matter surrounded by white matter. Fiber tracts traveling to and from the brain are found in the white matter. Also shown are the meningeal membranes (pia, arachnoid, and dura mater) that surround the spinal cord and are continuous with those surrounding the brain. The axons of the dorsal root ganglion neurons carry sensory information to the dorsal spinal cord through the dorsal root of the spinal nerve. Axons of the motor neurons in the ventral spinal cord leave through the ventral root. The fusion of these two roots forms the spinal nerve, which emerges from the vertebral column through an intervertebral foramen.

root contains the axons of motor neurons located in the ventral spinal cord. The two roots of each spinal nerve fuse before they exit the spinal canal through the particular intervertebral foramina that are associated with the spinal cord segment to which they are attached.

As in the brain, three protective layers called meninges cover the spinal cord. Tough and inflexible, the **dura mater** lines the skull and the vertebral canal. Lining the dura mater is the **arachnoid membrane**, which sends spidery, thin extensions of connective tissue called **arachnoid trabeculae** to the delicate **pia mater**, the layer that adheres to the surface of the spinal cord and the brain. Extensions from the pia mater anchor the spinal cord to the dura mater. Between the pia mater and the arachnoid layer is the **arachnoid space**. There, the cerebrospinal fluid flows around the brain and spinal cord. The cerebrospinal fluid is similar in composition to plasma, the fluid part of the blood.

Along with the optic and olfactory nerves and the 10 pairs of cranial nerves that exit the brainstem, the nerves (and their nerve roots) that exit the spinal cord are considered part of the peripheral nervous system. The peripheral nervous system has two divisions: the **somatic nervous system**, and the autonomic nervous system. Sensory neurons and their axons, as well as the axons of the motor neurons and preganglionic neurons located in the central nervous system, are all part of the peripheral nervous system.

If the spinal cord is cut in cross-section, you can see a butterfly-shaped area of gray matter around the small central spinal canal. Neurons that receive pain and sensory input are found in the dorsal "wings" of the butterfly; motor neurons that produce muscle movement are located in the ventral "wings." Surrounding the gray matter is the spinal cord's white matter. This consists of fiber tracts that run to and from the brain, as well as fibers that travel locally within a particular section of the spinal cord.

THE AUTONOMIC NERVOUS SYSTEM

The autonomic nervous system has three divisions: the **sympathetic nervous system**, the **parasympathetic nervous system**, and the **enteric nervous system**. The sympathetic nervous system makes energy available to the body during stress or emotional events. It produces the physiological changes that prepare the body for what is called the "fight or flight" response, in which the body gears up to either face or run away from danger. These changes include sweating, an increase in heart rate and blood pressure, a widening (dilation) of the pupils for better vision at a distance, a shifting of blood flow to the brain and muscles, and the activation of the adrenal medulla, which is considered a sympathetic ganglion because it develops from the neural crest.

The parasympathetic nervous system, on the other hand, has the opposite job: it conserves energy and helps the body return to normal after a stressful event. The parasympathetic nervous system serves a maintenance function. It is always working. The effects it produces on the body include an increase of blood flow to the intestines, slowing of the heart rate, and constriction of the pupils for closer vision. It brings the body functions back to normal after the sympathetic nervous system has been activated.

The enteric nervous system (ENS) consists of the neuronal networks, or plexi (singular is plexus) within the walls and underneath the lining of the gastrointestinal (GI) tract that operate independently of the central nervous system. There is communication back and forth between the brain and the ENS via the vagus nerve, but the ENS can perform its functions even if the vagus is cut. The ENS has its own sensory neurons, motor neurons, and interneurons, and uses a variety of neurotransmitters. It even sends nerves to the pancreas and gallbladder to help regulate their activities. The messages sent to the brain through the vagus nerve appear to have an effect on brain functions as well.

There are two types of neurons in the autonomic nervous system: preganglionic and postganglionic. Preganglionic neurons are located in the central nervous system in the motor nuclei of the cranial nerves and in the intermediolateral gray matter of the spinal cord. Their axons are called **preganglionic fibers**. Postganglionic neurons are found in ganglia, or groups of neurons, outside the central nervous system. (A collection of neurons with similar functions is called a ganglion if it is found in the peripheral nervous system, or a nucleus if it is part of the central nervous system.) The axons of postganglionic neurons are called **postganglionic fibers**.

Most of the postganglionic neurons of the sympathetic nervous system are located in a chain of sympathetic ganglia on either side of the spinal cord. As a result, their preganglionic fibers are much shorter than their postganglionic fibers, which synapse on their target organs. Postganglionic neurons of the parasympathetic nervous system are located on or close to their target organs. So their preganglionic fibers are very long, and their postganglionic fibers are short.

NEUROTRANSMITTERS

As we saw in Chapter 1, the neural signal has two components: an electrical signal that travels down the axon, and a chemical signal that crosses the synapse. For a neurochemical to be classified as a neurotransmitter, it has to meet certain criteria. It must be synthesized by the transmitting, or presynaptic, neuron and it must be stored inside presynaptic vesicles in the presynaptic terminal. A neurotransmitter must be released from the presynaptic terminal by mechanisms that require calcium ions to be present. These calcium ions enter the presynaptic terminal when the arrival of an action potential depolarizes it. The neurochemical must selectively activate specific receptors, causing a change in the membrane potential of the post-synaptic membrane. Finally, there have to be mechanisms in place by which the neurotransmitter is removed from the

synapse after release, either by reuptake (via specific transporters) into the presynaptic terminal or by being broken
down by specific enzymes in the postsynaptic membrane.
Dozens of neurochemicals meet all of these criteria.

Most neurotransmitters fall into one of four basic
groups, depending on their chemical structure: acetylcholine,
monoamines, amino acids, and peptides. Because its more
complex structure contains an amine group, acetylcholine
is sometimes placed with the monoamines into an "amine"
group. Table 3.4 contains a list of neurotransmitters in the
different groups. Neurotransmitters function by producing
depolarizing postsynaptic membrane potentials (excitatory)
or hyperpolarizing postsynaptic potentials (inhibitory). The
same neurotransmitter can have an excitatory effect when it
binds to one type of receptor and an inhibitory effect when
it binds to another type. Whether the effect is excitatory or
inhibitory depends on which ion channels are opened when the
neurotransmitter binds to the cell's receptors. If sodium ions
enter the cell, the postsynaptic membrane becomes depolarized.
Chloride ions and potassium ions, in contrast, have a hyperpolarizing effect on the postsynaptic membrane and, hence,
an inhibitory effect on the neuron's activity.

Acetylcholine

Acetylcholine was the first neurotransmitter to be discovered.
The presynaptic terminals of all motor neurons release acetylcholine. So do those of all autonomic preganglionic neurons, all
parasympathetic postganglionic neurons, and the sympathetic
postganglionic neurons that innervate the sweat glands.

Acetylcholine is made when an acetate molecule is
attached to a choline molecule by a reaction involving the
enzyme choline acetyltransferase. In the synapse, acetylcholine
is broken down (degraded) by acetylcholinesterase. There
are two types of acetylcholine (cholinergic) receptors:
nicotinic and muscarinic. Each of these has several subtypes.

Table 3.4 TRANSMITTERS IN THE HUMAN BRAIN

AMINES

Acetylcholine
Dopamine
Epinephrine
Histamine
Norepinephrine
Serotonin

AMINO ACIDS

Aspartate
Gamma-aminobutyric acid
Glycine
L-glutamate

NEUROPEPTIDES

Adrenocorticotrophic hormone (ACTH)
Adrenomedullin
Amylin
Angiotensin II
Apelin
Bradykinin
Calcitonin
Calcitonin gene-related peptide (CGRP)
Cholecystokinin (CCK)
Corticotropin releasing factor (CRF)
   (urocortin)
Dynorphins, neoendorphins
Endorphins, (lipotropic hormones [LPHs])
Endothelins
Enkephalins
Follicle stimulating hormone (FSH)
Galanin
Gastric inhibitory peptide (GIP)
Gastrin
Gastrin releasing peptide
Glucagon-like peptides (GLPs)
Gonadotropin releasing hormone (GnRH)

Growth hormone-releasing factor (GHRF)
Lipotropin hormone (LPH)
Luteinizing hormone (LH)
Melanin concentrating hormone (MCH)
Melanin stimulating hormone (MSH)
Motilin
Neurokinins
Neuromedins
Neurotensin (NT)
Neuropeptide FF (NPFF)
Neuropeptide Y (NPY)
Orexins/hypocretins
Orphanin
Oxytocin
Nociceptin/FG
Pituitary adenylate cyclase activating
   polypeptide (PACAP)
Pancreatic polypeptide (PP)
Peptide histidine isoleucine (PHI)
Parathyroid hormone (PTH)
Peptide YY (PYY)
Prolactin releasing peptide (PrRP)
Secretin/PHI
Somatostatin (SS) (cortistatin)
Tachykinins
Thyroid stimulating hormone (TSH)
Thyroid releasing hormone (TRH)
Urotensin II
Vasopressin
Vasoactive intestinal peptide (VIP)

OTHERS

Adenosine
Adenosine triphosphate
Anandamide (arachidonolyethanolamide)
Arachidonic acid
Nitric oxide

Nicotinic receptors are **ionotropic receptors.** That means that each receptor has a central ion channel that opens when the receptor is activated. Muscarinic receptors are **metabotropic receptors.** Instead of activating channels directly, they activate a special protein called G protein, a subunit of which either opens a channel directly by binding to it or indirectly by activating an enzyme that causes the synthesis of a **second messenger.** This second messenger then starts a series of biochemical events that results in the opening of ion channels. These extra steps make it take longer to initiate cellular events which involve metabotropic receptors.

Monoamines

The **monoamines** include dopamine, norepinephrine, epinephrine, and serotonin. Serotonin belongs to the indoleamine subclass, while the other three monoamines belong to the catecholamine subclass. The catecholamines are synthesized from the amino acid tyrosine in a series of enzymatic reactions that first produces L-DOPA, then dopamine, then norepinephrine, and finally epinephrine. **Monoamine oxidases** are enzymes that break down catecholamines. They are found in the blood and in catecholaminergic (activated by catecholamine) presynaptic terminals. All of the monoamines act on metabotropic receptors and release their transmitters from varicosities, or bead-like swellings on their axons, rather than at specific synapses.

Norepinephrine is produced and released by all post-ganglionic neurons of the sympathetic nervous system except those that innervate the sweat glands. Extensive projections from nuclei in the medulla, pons, and one thalamic region have an activating effect on other areas of the brain. They are also involved in appetite control and sexual behavior. The adrenal medulla makes and releases both norepinephrine and epinephrine into the bloodstream as hormones. These neurochemicals are an important part of the stress response, both as hormones and as neurotransmitters.

Dopamine may be either excitatory or inhibitory, depending on which of its receptor subtypes is activated. It is important in movement and the reward system. It is also involved in attention and learning. Some drugs (including cocaine, amphetamines, and methylphenidate) inhibit dopamine reuptake in the synapse and thereby increase the effects of dopamine.

Serotonin is involved in sleep, eating, arousal, dreaming, and the regulation of mood, body temperature, and pain transmission. It is made from the amino acid tryptophan by two enzymatic reactions. Hallucinogenic drugs produce their effects by stimulating a receptor in the forebrain that is sensitive to serotonin (serotonergic).

Amino Acids

Glutamate, also known as glutamic acid, is the most abundant excitatory neurotransmitter in the central nervous system. All incoming sensory endings in the nervous system use it to send their signals.

Gamma-amino butyric acid (GABA) is produced by the actions of enzymes on glutamic acid. GABA is believed to have sedative, anxiety-relieving, muscle-relaxing, and anticonvulsant effects. It also causes **amnesia**, or loss of memory, possibly because it inhibits the release of glutamate, which scientists believe is important in memory formation. It also inhibits the release of monoamines and acetylcholine, which facilitate the formation of memories by the brain.

Glycine is the simplest amino acid. It is concentrated in the spinal cord, medulla, and retina. Unlike other neurotransmitters, glycine is found only in animals with backbones (vertebrates) and humans. Neuroscientists currently know little about how glycine is made.

Both GABA and glycine help to maintain a balance in the nervous system. Although GABA is the main inhibitory transmitter in the brain, GABA and glycine are both important in the spinal cord. Left unchecked, glutamatergic excitatory transmission causes seizures and is neurotoxic (lethal to nerve cells). The lethal effects on cells of too much excitatory transmission and the free radicals that accompany it may be responsible for causing many diseases, such as cancer, inflammatory joint disease, diabetes, Parkinson's disease, and Alzheimer's disease. Free radicals have also been implicated in aging.

Neuropeptides

Neuropeptides are chains of linked amino acids that are produced in the brain. They are made from larger polypeptides that are cut into smaller segments by enzymes. There are three major groups of neuropeptides: **endogenous opioids**; peptides that are also found in the gastrointestinal tract (called gut peptides); and peptide hormones that the hypothalamus produces to control pituitary function. Many peptides are found in presynaptic terminals with other neurotransmitters and may help modulate the effects of the other transmitters.

The best known of the endogenous opioids are the enkephalins, which produce what is called the "runner's high"— the pleasurable feeling many athletes get from an intense workout. Other endogenous opioids are the endorphins and the dynorphins. There are several types of opioid receptors, all of which are metabotropic. When opioid receptors are activated, they cause **analgesia** (pain relief), **euphoria** (a feeling of extreme joy or elation), and also inhibit defensive responses such as hiding and fleeing. Synthetic (laboratory-produced) opiates and opiates that come from plants act on the receptors that produce euphoria. Because they cause feelings of pleasure, they help lead to **addiction** to certain drugs. Although highly addictive, opiates such as morphine are sometimes used in the medical setting for their painkilling effects.

Drug Effects

Many drugs produce their effects by interacting with neurotransmitter receptors or related synaptic mechanisms. Some, called **agonists**, actually mimic the effect of natural neuro-transmitters by binding to the receptor and activating it. The results are very similar to those that the neurotransmitter itself would have produced. Other drugs, called **antagonists**, bind to the receptor without activating it. This prevents the neuro-transmitter from binding to and activating the receptor. **Partial agonists** bind to the receptor and produce a smaller effect than the neurotransmitter itself. **Inverse agonists** bind to the receptor and produce an effect opposite to the one that is usually associated with the receptor.

CONNECTIONS

Protected by bone and three layers of meninges, the brain and spinal cord make up the central nervous system. The central, lateral, and parieto-occipital sulci form the boundaries of the four lobes of the cerebral hemispheres: frontal, parietal, temporal, and occipital. Six layers of neurons make up the gray matter of the cerebral cortex, and their axons form most of the underlying white matter. Nuclei at the base of the cerebrum overlie the diencephalon, which in turn lies on top of the brainstem. Fiber tracts descend through the midbrain, pons, and medulla on their way to the spinal cord, the nuclei in the brainstem, and the cerebellum, which overlies the fourth ventricle. The peripheral nervous system is made up of all the components of the nervous system located outside the brain and spinal cord, including the 12 pairs of cranial and 31 pairs of spinal nerves. The peripheral nervous system has two divisions: somatic and autonomic. Motor nerves that activate the skeletal muscles make up the somatic nervous system. Nerves of the autonomic nervous system regulate the viscera (internal organs) and the glands. The enteric nervous system regulates the movements of the gastrointestinal tract. Neuro-transmitters are the nervous system's chemical messengers. When they are released from the presynaptic terminals of neurons into the synaptic cleft, they bind to and activate postsynaptic receptors that are specific to each neurotransmitter. Glutamate is the most abundant excitatory neurotransmitter in the nervous system, and GABA is the major inhibitory neurotransmitter. Glycine is an important inhibitory neurotransmitter in the spinal cord. Acetylcholine, norepinephrine, dopamine, and serotonin increase the activation of parts of the cerebral cortex and also play roles in the sleep/wake cycle. Norepinephrine and epinephrine are important in the stress response, both as neurotransmitters and as hormones.

4

Sensation and Perception

In the autumn, we are awed by the dazzling array of colors the trees display as they prepare for the coming winter. In the winter, the intricate patterns of the snowflakes and the beauty of the blankets of snow amaze us. Spring and summer flowers, with their colors and aromas and the butterflies they attract, bring us pleasure. We listen to the birds singing in the trees and the sounds the wind makes as it rustles the leaves and grass. The ocean waves and their roar fill us with wonder as we walk along the beach and feel the sand beneath our feet. When we wade into the water, the tide tugs at our ankles as we enjoy the cool ocean breeze on our faces.

All of these experiences are made possible by our senses, which take in information about our environment and send it to our brains to be integrated and interpreted. **Sensation** refers to the process of receiving information through the sense organs. The sense organs detect chemical and physical stimuli in the environment. These stimuli cause changes in the sensory receptors. **Transduction** is the process by which physical or chemical stimuli are translated into neural signals by the sensory receptors. **Perception** refers to the process in which the brain combines, organizes, and interprets sensations.

The ancient Greek philosopher Aristotle (384–322 B.C.) described five senses: vision, hearing, smell, taste, and touch. Modern scientists recognize several other senses, too, including equilibrium, pressure, temperature, position sense, and pain. Each of the senses has its own receptors, sensory neurons, and neural pathways, which transmit the stimuli to specific targets in the brain. Sensory information may be processed at two or more different levels once it reaches the brain. We are not consciously aware of these processing stages, only of the resulting perception.

VISION

Much like a camera, the eye focuses incoming light rays on a thin membrane at the back of the eye called the **retina**, which might be compared to the film in the camera. Most of the eyeball is covered by a tough white membrane called the **sclera**. Between the sclera and the retina is a darkly pigmented layer filled with blood vessels. This layer is called the choroid. It provides nourishment to the retina. At the front of the eye, a transparent membrane called the **cornea** lets light into the eye. It is curved to help focus the incoming light rays.

Behind the cornea is the pigmented **iris**, which gives the eyes their color. The muscles in this circular structure can contract to widen (dilate) or relax to narrow (constrict) the **pupil**—the opening at the center of the iris. Light passes through the pupil and through the transparent **lens**, which focuses the light on the retina. Two muscles, one above and one below the lens, hold the lens in place and contract or relax to change the shape of the lens. The lens takes on a more spherical shape for near vision and a flatter shape for far vision.

The light reflected from an object is focused on the retina so that the image of the object is upside down and backward—much as it is on the film in a camera. The brain, however, reverses this image. In the space between the cornea and the lens, a fluid called **aqueous humor** circulates to provide nutrition to the cornea and lens, which have no blood vessels of their own. It also maintains pressure inside the eye. Behind the lens, the space inside the eye is filled with the **vitreous humor**, a gel-like substance that maintains the shape of the eyeball (Figure 4.1).

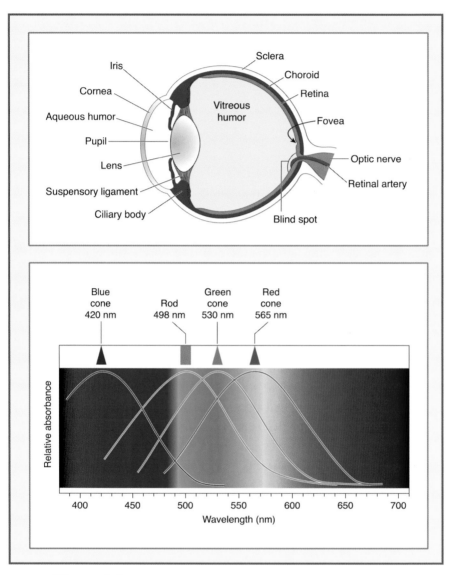

Figure 4.1 Our eyes are our "windows to the world." They are protected by the bony sockets in the skull called orbits. The structures of the human eye are shown in the top diagram. The human eye can detect electromagnetic radiation in wavelengths between 380 and 760 nm. This range of wavelengths is called the visible spectrum and falls between ultraviolet rays and infrared rays on the electromagnetic spectrum (bottom).

At the rear of the retina is a single layer of receptor cells that contain **photopigments**. These pigments go through chemical changes when they are exposed to light. These chemical changes cause ion channels in the cell membrane to open so that the receptor cell depolarizes and fires an action potential. Two layers of essentially transparent neurons lie in front of the pigmented **photoreceptor** layer. The neural signal generated by each photoreceptor cell goes to a **bipolar cell** in the layer closest to the photoreceptor layer. Each bipolar cell then sends the signal on to a **ganglion cell** in the retinal layer closest to the vitreous humor. Axons from the ganglion cells of each eye converge (come together) to form the optic nerve. The point at which the optic nerve leaves the eyeball on its way to the brain is called the "blind spot" because there are no photoreceptor cells there.

Named for their shapes, the eye's two types of receptor cells are called **rods** and **cones**. The eye has approximately 125 million rods and 6 million cones. Rods contain a pigment called rhodopsin, which is sensitive to as little as one photon of light. (A photon is the smallest unit of light at a particular wavelength.) This extreme sensitivity allows us to see in dim light. Rods also help the eyes detect movement.

The eye has three types of cones, each of which has one of three different color pigments. Each color pigment is most sensitive to one of three colors: red, blue, or green. The relative activity of the three different kinds of cones is important in determining the color-coding signal that goes to the brain.

Our visual acuity, or ability to see details, is greatest in bright light, when the cones are most active. It is poorest in dim light, when the rods are most active. In dim lighting, the edges of objects appear blurred, and we see in tones of gray rather than colors.

Light rays that enter the eye focus on the center of the retina in an area called the **macula**. It is here that the cones are most heavily concentrated. In the center of the macula is a tiny circular area about 1 mm in diameter (the size of a pinhead). This site, called the **fovea**, is indented because cone receptors are the only cells present there. The fovea is located just above the point where the optic nerve leaves the eye. Outside the macula, the concentration of cones begins to decrease, while the number of rods increases. The number of rods is greatest in an area that forms a circle at 20 degrees from the fovea in all directions. Vision is sharpest in the fovea. Vision loses its sharpness as the density of cones decreases farther away from the fovea.

As the two optic nerves exit behind the eyes, they travel medially (toward the center) to the **optic chiasm**, just in front of the hypothalamus. There, the axons of the ganglion cells in the half of the retina closest to the nose (the nasal half) on each

WHAT IS COLOR BLINDNESS?

Color blindness is the inability to distinguish between either red and green (most common) or yellow and blue. An absence of all color, when a person sees only in tones of gray, is very rare. The genes for the pigments of the red and green cones lie close together on the X chromosome, of which females have two copies and males have only one. Since color blindness is a recessive trait, a female would have to have defective genes on both X chromosomes for the trait to be expressed. Because this is unlikely, only about 0.4% of females are color-blind, whereas approximately 8% of males are.

The gene for the blue pigment is found on chromosome 7, of which both sexes have two copies. As a result, this type of color blindness is less common, affecting about 1 person in 10,000.

If the gene for one of the visual color pigments is defective or missing, that pigment will be expressed in lower quantities in the cones of the retina or not expressed at all. As a result, the color-blind person will see the world in shades and combinations of the two color pigments that are expressed.

side cross and travel toward the opposite, or **contralateral**, side of the brain. The axons of the ganglion cells in the half of the retina closest to the temple (the temporal half) do not cross. Instead, they travel toward the same, or **ipsilateral**, side of the brain. Because of this, neural signals from both eyes that contain visual information from the left side of the visual field end up on the right side of the brain, and vice versa.

From the optic chiasm, 90% of the fibers on each side travel to the **lateral geniculate nucleus** of the thalamus on the same side and synapse on neurons there. From this relay nucleus in the thalamus, the visual information is sent to the primary visual cortex. It is here that visual information is processed and relayed to the rest of the brain. All sensory inputs except olfactory (smell) go first to the thalamus before the signals travel to the cerebral cortex. The other 10% of fibers reach other targets on that side.

Axons from each lateral geniculate nucleus travel as an **optic radiation** through the temporal lobe back to the ipsilateral **primary visual cortex**, most of which is folded into the **calcarine fissure** at the pole of the occipital lobe. The **secondary visual cortex**, where processing of raw visual data begins, surrounds the primary visual cortex around the outside of the calcarine fissure. Projections from the visual cortex reach other areas of the cortex, allowing visual information to be integrated with information from the other senses. It is estimated that in humans, 25 to 40% of the cerebral cortex plays some role in the processing of visual information.

Vision loss that results from damage to the central pathways varies with the specific location of the damage (lesion). If one optic nerve is completely cut, there will be blindness in the ipsilateral eye. Partial damage to the optic nerve causes a small blind spot called a scotoma. A person with this problem may not even notice it if it affects only the peripheral visual field. However, if it affects the fovea, there will be a noticeable reduction in the sharpness of vision. Damage to the optic chiasm, which often occurs as a result of pituitary tumors, causes a bilateral loss of the temporal half of the visual field. This affects peripheral vision. Again, the sufferer may not realize there is a problem unless he or she has an accident because of the peripheral vision loss.

AUDITORY SENSE (HEARING)

The many sounds in our environment range from the quiet tick of a clock to the roar of a jet engine or a clap of thunder. Sound waves travel through the air at 700 miles (1,127 kilometers) per hour to our ears (Figure 4.2). They are funneled by the **pinna**— the external flap of skin and cartilage that we think of when the word *ear* comes to mind—into the ear canal. At the end of the ear canal is a thin membrane called the **tympanic membrane**, or **eardrum**. All of these structures together make up what is known as the **outer ear**. When sound waves reach the eardrum, they make it vibrate. These vibrations are transmitted across the air-filled space of the **middle ear** by means of three tiny bones, or **ossicles**. These bones are named for their shapes: the *malleus* (hammer), *incus* (anvil), and *stapes* (stirrup). The malleus is attached to the eardrum, and the stapes is attached to the membrane that covers the inside of the oval window, an opening in the fluid-filled **cochlea**, or inner ear. Opposite the cochlea, there is a set of bony canals that are involved in our sense of balance.

Sound waves produced by the vibration of objects in our environment are detected by the human ear in the range of 30 to 20,000 vibrations per second. Unlike the eye, which combines wavelengths to produce the perception of a single color, the ear does not combine the frequencies it receives, but hears them as separate tones. Since most of us cannot move our ears, we turn our heads to hear better, an action which allows the outer ear to be a more efficient "sound funnel." Tiny muscles attached to the stapes and malleus react reflexively to loud noises by contracting, causing the chain of ossicles to

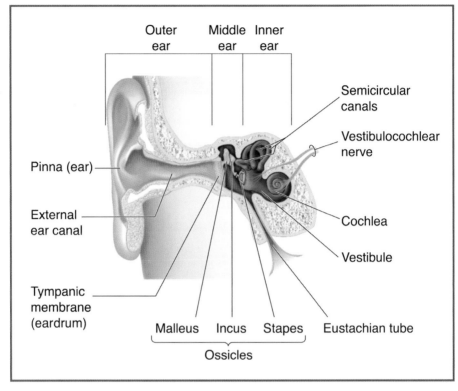

Figure 4.2 The human ear, illustrated here, is composed of three regions: the outer, middle, and inner ears. Sound waves produced by the vibrations of objects in the environment enter the outer ear, and strike the eardrum, which separates the outer ear from the middle ear. These sound waves cause the eardrum to vibrate, and the vibrations are then transmitted to the inner ear via the ossicles. It is in the cochlea of the inner ear that these vibrations are transduced (turned into) electrical impulses, which are then sent to the brain for interpretation.

stiffen and the eardrum to become more taut. This results in less low frequency sound being transmitted by the ossicles and more being reflected by the eardrum. It is thought that this helps protect the ear from damage. Some scientists think that the reflex selectively filters low-frequency transmission to reduce background "noise" and hear meaningful sounds better.

The cochlea is a bony structure that resembles a snail in shape. It contains the receptor cells and auditory neurons that collect sound wave data and convert it into neural signals. If the "coil" of the cochlea were straightened out, we would see two membranes extending the length of the coil. The lower, flexible membrane is called the basilar membrane. Embedded in this basilar membrane are hair cells. These are the receptors for the **auditory**, or hearing, sense. Suspended above the basilar membrane is the rigid tectorial membrane. Together, the basilar membrane, tectorial membrane, and hair cells make up what is called the **organ of Corti**.

As the oval window vibrates in response to the movement of the stapes against it, the fluid that fills the cochlea and circulates around the basilar membrane moves. This, in turn, causes the basilar membrane to vibrate. Hair-like structures called cilia at the tip of each hair cell are embedded in the tectorial membrane. As the basilar membrane moves, these cilia bend. This causes potassium ion channels in the hair cell to open and generate an action potential.

Because they have no axons, auditory hair cells synapse directly on the dendrites of bipolar neurons whose axons form the cochlear nerve, which merges with the auditory nerve. Neurotransmitter molecules released from the bases of the hair cells transmit the signal by binding to receptors on the auditory neurons. The pathway of the auditory neural signal to the brain is complex. It branches several times to synapse on structures along the way. As a result, each structure in this complicated pathway receives auditory information from both ears. One of these structures is the **medial geniculate nucleus**, which is located in the thalamus. From the medial geniculate nuclei, the auditory information is transmitted to the primary auditory cortex, which is found in the posterior superior temporal lobe at the edge of and extending into the lateral fissure. Projections from the primary auditory cortex go to the surrounding secondary auditory cortex. The higher-order auditory cortex surrounds the secondary auditory cortex and extends laterally to the edge of the superior temporal sulcus. Processing of auditory information is hierarchical, in that the processing of sounds, ranging from simple tones to speech perception, becomes increasingly complex at each ascending level. Projections from the auditory association cortex to the polymodal cortex, which lies inside the superior temporal sulcus, allow the integration of auditory information with visual information and information from the body senses. As with visual information, auditory information reaches multiple areas of the cortex for integration with other sensory information.

In the left temporal lobe, there is an area of the higher-order auditory cortex known as **Wernicke's area**, or speech receptive area. If this area is damaged, the person experiences a loss of speech *comprehension,* or the ability to understand speech. The equivalent area in the right temporal lobe interprets emotional aspects of language. Other higher-order auditory areas extend from the temporal lobe up into the lower parietal lobe. They are important in writing and reading. Projections from auditory primary and secondary areas go to **Broca's area**, or the motor speech area, located on the other side of the lateral fissure in the lower frontal lobe on the left side of the brain. Damage to this area results in an impairment of speech *production.* That is, speech becomes garbled or, with severe damage, completely absent.

Approximately 10% of adults suffer from some degree of deafness (loss of hearing). There are two basic types of deafness. Conductive deafness involves the middle ear or the outer ear canal. The most common causes are an overaccumulation of earwax (cerumen) or an inflammation in the middle ear. Otosclerosis is a less common form of conductive deafness. In this condition, the joint between the vestibule of the inner ear and the footplate of the stapes becomes rigid and bony (calcifies), making the stapes unable to move. Sensorineural deafness usually results when the neurons in the inner ear degenerate. This type of deafness can be caused by a noisy work environment, mumps or German measles infections, a tumor, or certain drugs (particularly antibiotics).

EQUILIBRIUM (BALANCE)

Our sense of balance is called the vestibular sense. It is regulated by the vestibular system. The vestibular organs are part of the inner ear. Vestibular receptors are found in three semicircular canals opposite the cochlea, and also in two saclike structures called the utricle and saccule that are located next to the cochlea in the **vestibule**. The cilia of the vestibular receptor cells are embedded in a gel-like mass called the cupula, which covers the hair cells. When our head turns, the movement of the fluid in the semicircular canals displaces the gelatinous mass, making the cilia bend. In the saccule and utricle, calcium carbonate crystals within the gelatinous mass lie on top of the cilia. When the head moves forward, these crystals move and bend the cilia, sending signals to the brain about the change in the head's position.

Sensory pathways that go up from the vestibular nuclei help control neck and head position by sending the brain information about body and visual orientation. Vestibular sensory information goes first to the ventral posterior nuclei of the thalamus and from there to the parietal lobe and the insula. Two motor pathways go down from the vestibular nuclei to the spinal cord. One of these pathways, the lateral vestibulospinal tract, reaches neurons in the spinal cord at all levels. It is crucial in the control of balance and posture. The other pathway, called the medial vestibulospinal tract, travels to the cervical and upper thoracic areas of the spinal cord and helps control head position. Other fibers from the vestibular nuclei go to the cerebellum, the reticular formation, the motor nuclei that control the eye muscles, and back to the vestibular organ itself. Projections to the oculomotor nuclei cause reflex adjustments of eye movements as the head moves. If the vestibular system malfunctions, we can experience vertigo (dizziness) and problems with balance.

GUSTATION (TASTE)

Taste and smell are known as the chemical senses because their receptors respond to chemical stimuli. All of the other senses respond to physical stimuli. Our sense of taste serves two important functions: to meet our nutritional needs by detecting food molecules dissolved in saliva, and to detect poisons in ingested substances. There are a few basic taste qualities: sweet, salty, sour, and bitter. There is also a fifth taste quality called *umami* (Japanese for "delicious") that has recently been identified. (Umami is the taste quality associated with the amino acid glutamate and salts of glutamate, such as monosodium glutamate, or MSG.) A particular flavor is a combination of one or more of the five basic taste qualities. Taste and smell both contribute to our perception of flavor. In fact, smell plays the greater role. You can find this out for yourself. Try holding your nose while tasting some familiar foods. How do they taste now?

Altogether, there are about 10,000 **taste buds** on the surface of the tongue, roof of the mouth, pharynx, epiglottis, larynx, and upper esophagus (Figure 4.3). Most of these taste buds are associated with the taste papillae (singular is *papilla*) that appear as tiny red bumps on the surface of the tongue. All taste buds can detect all five taste qualities. Some, however, are more sensitive to one taste quality than to the others. Hence, a simplistic "taste map" of the tongue shows the tip of the tongue as more sensitive to sweet and salty tastes, the sides of the tongue to sour tastes, and the back of the tongue and back of the mouth to bitter tastes.

Each taste bud is an onion-shaped cluster of about 100 taste receptor cells. These structures do the actual work of detecting taste sensations. Each of these cells lives for about 1 to 2 weeks before dying and being replaced. From 3 to 250 taste buds can be found on the sides or top of each taste papilla. Fibers from

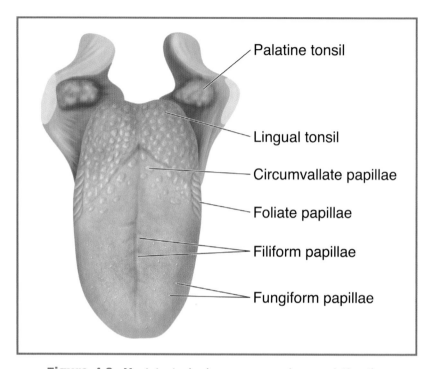

Palatine tonsil

Lingual tonsil

Circumvallate papillae

Foliate papillae

Filiform papillae

Fungiform papillae

Figure 4.3 Most taste buds are arranged around the tiny papillae or "bumps" on the surface of the tongue. They are found in the moat-like trenches of the circumvallate papillae, inside the folds of the foliate papillae, and on the surface of the mushroom-shaped fungiform papillae. Filiform papillae, which are shaped like cones, are the most numerous but do not contain taste buds. Although fewer in number than the other papillae, the circumvallate papillae contain almost half of the approximately 5,000 taste buds on the tongue.

three cranial nerves connect to the taste buds. Fibers carrying taste information travels to the solitary nucleus in the medulla, where they synapse on neurons that send taste information to the ipsilateral ventral posterior medial nucleus of the thalamus. (Some fibers that leave the solitary nucleus travel to motor nuclei of cranial nerves. These participate in coughing and swallowing and other reflexes related to taste.) Taste information is then relayed from the thalamus to the **insular**

cortex and frontal lobe operculum. (The **insula** can be seen at the floor of the lateral fissure by pulling back the overlying edges, or opercula, of the temporal and frontal lobes.) Information from the gustatory cortex goes to the orbital cortex in the frontal lobe for integration with olfactory information and to the amygdala, from which the information is relayed to the hypothalamus and other areas associated with learning and memory.

As we get older, the number of taste receptors we have gradually declines. The sense of taste can be impaired by smoking, gingivitis, strep throat, influenza, a lack of vitamin B_{12} or zinc, side effects of certain drugs, or injuries to the head or mouth. A partial loss of the sense of taste is called **hypogeusia**. The total loss of all taste sensation is called **ageusia**.

OLFACTION (SMELL)

Airborne molecules are detected by **olfactory receptors**— proteins that span the membranes of the cilia of **primary olfactory neurons** in the lining of the nasal cavity. There are about 5 million of these neurons in each nostril, residing in two patches that are each a few centimeters square and located directly below the eyes. Primary olfactory neurons live for about a month before they are replaced by neurons that develop from stem cells known as basal cells. There are about 1,000 types of olfactory receptors, which together can detect up to 10,000 different odors. However, only one type of receptor appears on any given olfactory neuron.

Primary olfactory neuronal axons travel up through tiny openings in the **cribriform plate** to synapse in clusters on the paired olfactory bulbs on the underside of the frontal lobe. Axons from the olfactory bulb neurons travel through the **olfactory tract** to the ipsilateral primary olfactory cortex, which includes the olfactory nucleus, the amygdala, and areas in the temporal lobe and ventral frontal cortex. Some of these structures play a role in emotion regulation and memory.

Unlike sensory information that comes from the other sense organs, smell signals travel first to the primary olfactory cortex before going to subcortical structures, such as the thalamus. However, olfactory messages go to the dorsomedial nucleus of the thalamus on their way from the primary olfactory cortex to the orbital cortex and adjacent insula, where the secondary olfactory cortex is located near the gustatory cortex (Figure 4.4).

Viruses, some medications, head injuries, and chemicals such as insecticides, chlorine, benzene, and mercury can destroy primary olfactory neurons in the nasal cavity. We also gradually lose some of our sense of smell as we age. Early symptoms of Parkinson's disease and Alzheimer's disease include a loss of smell sensation. A complete loss of the sense of smell is called **anosmia**, whereas a partial loss is called **hyposmia**.

SOMATOSENSES (BODY SENSES)

The cell bodies of the neurons that receive information from the body senses—including touch, pressure, vibration, pain, sense of position, and awareness of movement—are found in sense organs and **ganglia**, or clusters of neurons, in the brainstem and near the spinal cord. Their axons leave the brainstem as the sensory component of certain cranial nerves and the spinal cord as the sensory component of the spinal nerves. Cranial nerves that supply the skin, muscles, and other tissues of the face and neck have sensory fibers that carry information from somatosensory receptors to the brain as well as motor fibers that bring movement-related commands to muscles. Each dorsal root ganglion neuron of the spinal cord has an axonal process that enters the spinal cord and synapses on spinal cord neurons, and also has a long dendritic process that reaches to the peripheral organs and tissues.

Surrounding each peripheral nerve is a three-layered sheath of connective tissue that is continuous with the meninges of the brain and spinal cord. Around some

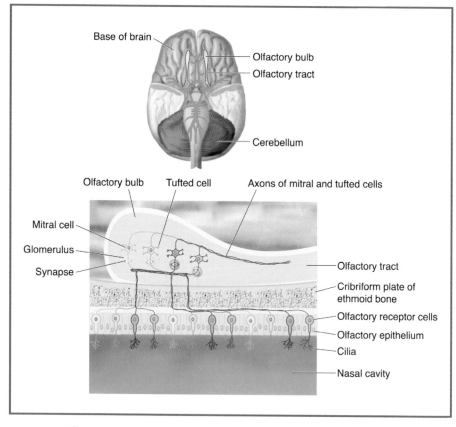

Figure 4.4 The axons of olfactory neurons travel in small bundles up through tiny openings in the cribriform ("perforated") plate of the ethmoid bone to synapse on neurons in the olfactory bulb. Axon terminals of olfactory neurons and dendrites of olfactory bulb neurons (mitral and tufted cells) and interneurons (periglomerular cells) form a structure called a glomerulus. The axons of the mitral cells and tufted cells travel from the olfactory bulb through the olfactory tract to the primary olfactory cortex.

somatosensory nerve endings is a capsule (sheath). Depending on the type of receptor, the capsule is part of either the outer layer (which is continuous with the dura mater) or the middle layer (which is continuous with the arachnoid membrane). These nerve endings are said to be *encapsulated* somatosensory receptors. Some nerve ending capsules are thin. Others are layered, some elaborately so. All nerve endings are covered with the nerve sheath's inner layer, which is continuous with the pia mater. Nerve endings that have no capsule are called **free nerve endings,** or *unencapsulated* somatosensory receptors.

Free nerve endings are found in the skin, in the pulp around the teeth, in the muscles and internal organs, and in the membranes that cover the muscles, bones, joints, organs, and line the body cavity. Depending on where they are located, these tiny branching dendritic ends can turn mechanical (touch, pressure, vibration, stretch), thermal (temperature), chemical (prostaglandins), and pain stimuli into neural signals.

Free nerve endings in the skin wrap around the bases of individual hairs and are activated when the hairs bend. Disk-shaped encapsulated **Merkel endings** are found in the basal layer of the epidermis (the outer layer of the skin). They are found in places like fingertips that need a fine sense of touch. **Meissner's corpuscles** with elongated capsules are found just below the epidermis. They, too, are especially abundant in the fingertips, and respond strongly to light touch. **Pacinian corpuscles** are found just beneath the skin and in other connective tissues, including muscles and joints. They look like an onion in cross-section. They are sensitive to pressure. **Ruffini's corpuscles,** which sense stretch, have cigar-shaped capsules. They are found in the dermis (the skin layer beneath the epidermis) as well as in other connective tissue. It is due to Meissner's and Merkel receptors that we have such excellent ability to tell the difference between items by touching them. Pacinian corpuscles are especially good at detecting vibrations.

In addition to having many free nerve endings, muscle tissue has two specialized encapsulated receptors: the **muscle spindles** and the **Golgi tendon organs.** Muscle spindles are scattered throughout all of our skeletal muscles. These long, thin stretch receptors are made up of a few muscle fibers with a capsule around the middle third of the structure. Muscle fibers involved in skeletal movement are called **extrafusal muscle fibers**. Attached at their ends to the extrafusal muscle fibers, the fibers of the muscle spindles are called **intrafusal muscle fibers**. When an extrafusal muscle is extended, the muscle spindles are stretched. This causes ion channels to open and generate a neural signal.

The muscle spindles detect changes in muscle length, whereas Golgi tendon organs detect muscle tension. Found at the point where tendons and muscles meet, these spindle-shaped receptors are similar in structure to Ruffini's corpuscles. Surprisingly, research has shown that it is the muscle spindles—not the Golgi tendon organs—that are more important in **proprioreception**, our sense of body position, and in **kinesthesia**, the sense that makes us aware of our body movements.

Pain receptors (**nociceptors**) detect intense or painful stimuli. These stimuli may be mechanical (cutting or pinching), thermal (cold or hot), or chemicals that the body releases into damaged tissue. Individual nociceptors may detect only one of these stimuli, or they may detect all three. Nociceptors are present in the skin, the membranes around bones, muscle sheaths, artery walls, the dura mater, and the membranes that cover and line internal organs and body cavities.

Nociceptors are the free nerve endings of pain fibers. These nerve endings can be further sensitized by chemicals released into the tissues after injury. This may explain why injured areas, such as sunburned skin, are sensitive to touch. There are no pain receptors in the brain itself or in the actual tissues of the internal organs. Because of this unique fact, patients are often kept awake during brain surgery, since they feel no pain from the procedure.

Two types of fibers branch into the free nerve endings that are nociceptors and are associated with two different types of pain. A-delta fibers, which are small in diameter and thinly myelinated, are responsible for "fast pain"—the sharp, stabbing pain that immediately alerts the body that an injury has occurred. C fibers, which are very small and unmyelinated, send their signals more slowly. They are responsible for slow, recurring, or aching pain.

Signals from both types of pain fibers travel first to the spinal cord, where the axons of the dorsal root ganglion neurons synapse on neurons in the dorsal horns of the spinal cord gray matter. Axons from the pain neurons in the spinal cord cross to the contralateral side and then travel up the spinal cord to the brainstem in the lateral spinothalamic tract, a pathway located in the lateral white matter of the spinal cord. Fibers from thermal receptors also travel in the lateral spinothalamic tract.

Pain information from C fibers takes a slow route through the reticular formation in the medulla and pons to the thalamus and hypothalamus and other areas that connect with the amygdala and hypothalamus. This means that the pain signals are sent to a widespread network. Since areas such as the amygdala and hypothalamus are involved in emotion, some of these pathways may be involved in the emotions that are often associated with pain.

CONNECTIONS

Information transduced from internal and environmental stimuli by sensory receptors travels through dendritic fibers to the dorsal root ganglia and the sensory nuclei of the cranial nerves. Except for olfactory information, sensory signals go to the thalamus before being transmitted to the appropriate primary sensory cortices. Olfactory information goes to the primary olfactory cortex before it is relayed through the thalamus to the secondary olfactory cortex. The thalamic relay nuclei for the senses are the lateral geniculate nucleus for vision, the medial geniculate nucleus for hearing, the dorsomedial nucleus for olfaction (smell), the ventral posterior nucleus for the vestibular sense, the ventral posterior medial nucleus for taste and the somatosenses, and the ventral posteriolateral nucleus for pain.

The primary sensory cortex, where raw sensory data is interpreted, is found in the calcarine fissure for vision, inside the lateral sulcus for hearing, in the insula and parietal cortex for balance, in the insula and frontal operculum for taste, in the insula and cingulate cortex for pain, in the somatosensory cortex for the body senses other than pain, and in several anterior temporal areas for smell. Secondary sensory cortex is located around the outside of the calcarine fissure for vision, in the orbitofrontal cortex for taste and smell, in the lateral sulcus surrounding and posterior to its primary sensory area for hearing, and in the insular cortex and parietal operculum for the somatosenses. Higher-order centers process information of increasing complexity and integrate information from the different sensory modalities.

5

Movement

Most of the interactions we have with our physical and social environments involve movement. During the developmental milestones of infancy, we develop the ability to make simple movements such as looking, speaking, reaching, walking, or running. More complex movements—for example, typing, skiing, riding a bicycle, dancing, playing a musical instrument, or drawing—must be learned, but the individual steps you need to make the movements become automatic over time. Our nervous system controls all of these different kinds of movement through a complex set of interactions between the motor areas of the brain, the spinal cord, and the nerves and fiber pathways that connect them to each other and to the muscles (Figure 5.1).

MUSCLE TYPES

Our bodies have three basic types of muscles: skeletal (or striated) muscle; smooth muscle; and cardiac muscle. **Skeletal muscles** are usually attached to two different bones—one at each end. When these muscles contract, they move the bones of the limbs and other areas. **Smooth muscles** in the eye control the size of the pupil and the shape of the lens. There are also smooth muscles around the hair follicles, in the sphincters of the urinary bladder and anus, and in the walls of the blood vessels and the digestive, urinary, and reproductive tracts. **Cardiac muscle** is found only in the walls of the heart. Although it looks somewhat like striated muscle, it functions more like smooth muscle.

Smooth muscle is under the control of the autonomic nervous system, which is controlled by the hypothalamus. Smooth muscle and cardiac muscle are sometimes called **involuntary** muscles because they usually function automatically, without our conscious control. Skeletal muscle, on the other hand, is often described as **voluntary**, since we consciously control most of our skeletal movements. Some movements of skeletal muscles, however, are involuntary responses (**reflexes**) to certain stimuli, particularly stimuli that signal danger. For example, when your hand jerks away from a hot stove, your muscles have responded reflexively to the danger—the heat that might burn your hand.

The synapse between an ending of an alpha motor neuron and a muscle fiber is called a **neuromuscular junction**, and the postsynaptic membrane of the synapse is a specialized area of the muscle membrane called the **muscle endplate**. Muscle endplates contain nicotinic receptors. Each muscle fiber has one muscle endplate surrounded by a Schwann cell to keep the neurotransmitter molecules inside the synapse.

ANATOMY AND PHYSIOLOGY OF THE NEUROMUSCULAR SYSTEM

A muscle fiber is a bundle of **myofibrils**, which are made up of strands, or filaments, of myosin and actin molecules. These filaments interact to make muscles contract. The **striations** of skeletal muscles are the dark stripes formed where filaments of myosin and actin overlap. Each motor neuron sends out an axon through the ventral, or motor, root of the spinal cord or out from the brainstem (in the case of cranial nerves) to the muscle fibers that it synapses on and activates. The number of muscle fibers a particular motor neuron stimulates depends on how coarse or fine the movements involved are. The branched endings of a motor neuron may activate as many as 1,000 fibers in the large muscles of the thigh and hip, while another motor neuron may stimulate fewer than 10 fibers in the muscles of the fingers, where more precise movements are required. Since a motor neuron has to send neural signals to fewer fibers in the fingers,

(continued on page 76)

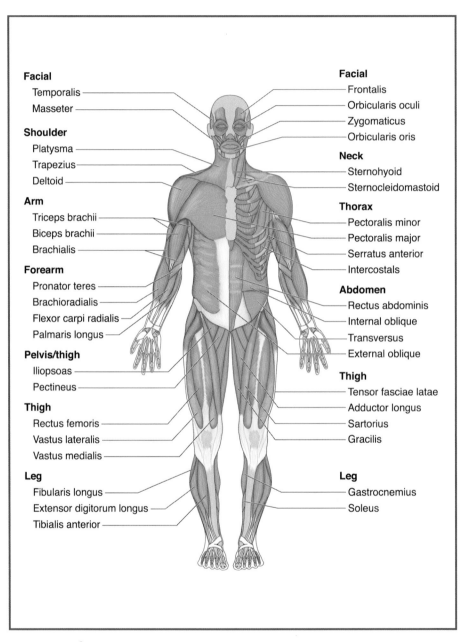

Facial
Temporalis
Masseter

Shoulder
Platysma
Trapezius
Deltoid

Arm
Triceps brachii
Biceps brachii
Brachialis

Forearm
Pronator teres
Brachioradialis
Flexor carpi radialis
Palmaris longus

Pelvis/thigh
Iliopsoas
Pectineus

Thigh
Rectus femoris
Vastus lateralis
Vastus medialis

Leg
Fibularis longus
Extensor digitorum longus
Tibialis anterior

Facial
Frontalis
Orbicularis oculi
Zygomaticus
Orbicularis oris

Neck
Sternohyoid
Sternocleidomastoid

Thorax
Pectoralis minor
Pectoralis major
Serratus anterior
Intercostals

Abdomen
Rectus abdominis
Internal oblique
Transversus
External oblique

Thigh
Tensor fasciae latae
Adductor longus
Sartorius
Gracilis

Leg
Gastrocnemius
Soleus

Figure 5.1 Our muscles produce all of our movements, both voluntary and involuntary. The skeletal, or voluntary, muscles of the human body are illustrated here.

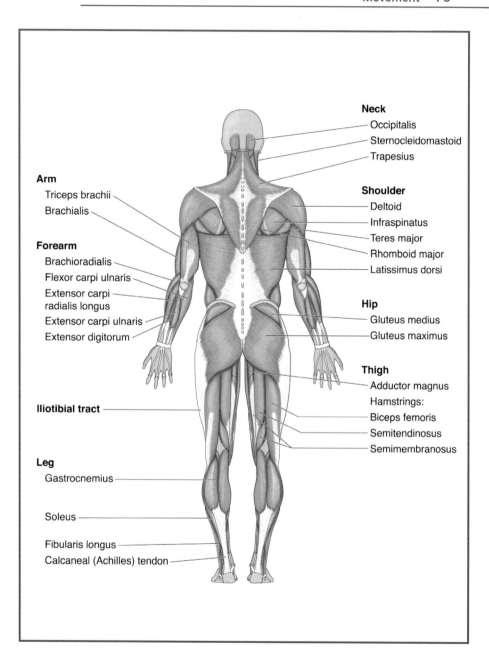

Neck
Occipitalis
Sternocleidomastoid
Trapesius

Arm
Triceps brachii
Brachialis

Shoulder
Deltoid
Infraspinatus
Teres major
Rhomboid major
Latissimus dorsi

Forearm
Brachioradialis
Flexor carpi ulnaris
Extensor carpi
radialis longus
Extensor carpi ulnaris
Extensor digitorum

Hip
Gluteus medius
Gluteus maximus

Thigh
Adductor magnus
Hamstrings:
Biceps femoris
Semitendinosus
Semimembranosus

Iliotibial tract

Leg
Gastrocnemius

Soleus

Fibularis longus
Calcaneal (Achilles) tendon

(continued from page 73)

these signals can be more specific than those for thigh muscles, for example. A **motor unit** consists of a motor neuron, its axon and nerve endings, and the set of muscle fibers that it activates.

A skeletal muscle is made up of a large group—that may include several hundreds—of parallel muscle fibers. Usually, it attaches at its opposite ends to two bones by bands of connective tissues called tendons. There is often a joint between the two bones. Some muscles make a limb bend (flex); these kinds of muscles are called **flexors**. Other muscles cause a limb to straighten out (extend); these are called **extensors**. For every flexor muscle, there is an opposing extensor muscle. This rule also applies to muscles that attach to only one bone, such as the muscles of the eye and tongue. Sometimes groups of muscles attach across a joint and work as a group; these are known as **synergistic** muscles. In such cases, there is one group of synergistic flexor muscles and an opposing synergistic group of extensor muscles.

NERVOUS SYSTEM CONTROL OF MOVEMENT

Motor commands travel from the motor cortex down to the cranial nerve nuclei or the spinal cord and out to the muscle fibers. So let us start in the brain and move downward as we look at the ways that the nervous system controls and coordinates muscle movements.

Cerebral Cortex

Several areas of the cerebral cortex are important in movement control (Figure 5.2). In the frontal lobe in front of the central sulcus is the precentral gyrus. This is where the primary motor cortex is located. Studies of the brain have shown that every area of the body is represented here. Those parts of the body that perform finer movements, such as the lips and fingers, are much more heavily represented.

The three main movement-related areas of the cortex are the premotor cortex, the supplementary motor cortex, and the

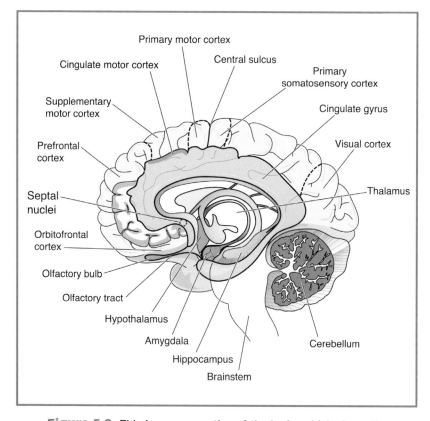

Figure 5.2 This is a cross-section of the brain, which shows the medial portions of the primary and supplementary motor cortices. Notice that the secondary motor cortex is located in the frontal lobe rostral to the primary motor cortex. The primary motor cortex is located in the precentral gyrus rostral to the central sulcus. In this view, the cingulate motor cortex and the supplementary motor cortex are visible. On the lateral aspect of the hemisphere, the supplementary motor cortex extends for a short distance and then the premotor cortex extends down to the temporal lobe.

cingulate motor area. The premotor cortex helps control our voluntary response to stimuli. The cingulate motor area is part of the **limbic system** (which is involved in the regulation of emotions). This part of the cortex may be involved in motor responses to drives and emotions. The supplementary motor cortex helps plan voluntary movements, as opposed to movements made in response to a stimulus.

DESCENDING PATHWAYS

Two main groups of fiber highways carry signals from the brain to the motor neurons that control muscle contractions. The lateral group descends through the white matter lateral to the spinal cord gray matter, whereas the ventromedial group travels in the ventromedial (ventral and adjacent to the midline) white matter of the spinal cord. While the ventromedial group synapses on the motor neurons in the ventromedial gray matter, the lateral group synapses on motor neurons in the lateral ventral gray matter. Neural signals that travel down the lateral pathways control and regulate voluntary movements of the limbs and extremities. Ventromedial pathways regulate posture by controlling trunk muscles and limb muscles close to the trunk.

About 1 million fibers descend together from the primary and secondary motor cortex in the **corticospinal tract**. Just above the juncture of the medulla and spinal cord, about 80% of these fibers cross to the opposite side of the medulla. They continue down the spinal cord as the lateral corticospinal tract. Another 10% do not cross but travel down the lateral corticospinal tract ipsilaterally. The remaining 10% of uncrossed fibers travel as the ventral corticospinal tract in the ventral or anterior white matter. They cross to the other side of the spinal cord as they reach their targets in the cervical and upper thoracic spinal cord. Fibers of the **corticobulbar tract** leave the motor cortices and travel ventral to the corticospinal tract until they reach their targets: cranial nerve motor neurons and associated interneurons in the reticular formation. Through the corticobulbar tract, the cerebral cortex exerts control over movements of the muscles of the face and head.

The other descending motor pathways start in the brainstem. Fibers of the **rubrospinal tract** begin in the red nucleus, which is located in the ventral midbrain at the same level as the superior colliculus. Rubrospinal tract fibers cross immediately to the contralateral side of the midbrain before descending through the brainstem and down the lateral white matter of the spinal cord. Fibers of the **vestibulospinal tract**, which originate in the vestibular nuclei (located in the pons and medulla), travel uncrossed down the spinal cord in the ventromedial white matter. Most fibers of the **tectospinal tract**, which begins in the superior colliculus of the midbrain, cross close to their point of origin and travel down the contralateral brainstem and the contralateral ventromedial white matter of the spinal cord. **Reticulospinal tract** fibers originate from the reticular formation in the pons and medulla. Those from the pons descend uncrossed in the ventromedial white matter of the spinal cord. Reticulospinal fibers that start in the medulla may be crossed or uncrossed and go down through the lateral white matter of the spinal cord. Scientists believe that fibers of the autonomic nervous system descend with the reticulospinal fibers.

Motor neurons in the ventrolateral spinal cord that innervate the limbs and extremities are the main targets of the fibers of the lateral corticospinal tract, which is important in independent movements of the fingers and in skilled, rapid movements of the hands. Ending primarily in the ventrolateral gray matter of the cervical spinal cord, the rubrospinal tract is thought to be important in the control of movements of hand and arm muscles but not independent finger movements. Ending on motor neurons in the ventromedial gray matter of the ipsilateral cervical and thoracic spinal cord, the ventral corticospinal tract helps control movements of the upper trunk muscles, the shoulders, and the neck. The tectospinal tract, which projects to the cervical spinal cord, is also involved in controlling trunk, shoulder, and neck movements, especially reflexive responses to auditory, visual, and possibly somatosensory stimuli.

Since the superior colliculus is important in the control of eye movements, part of the function of the tectospinal tract may be to coordinate head and eye movements. Descending primarily through the ipsilateral spinal cord, the reticulospinal tracts are involved in the control of automatic movements and functions that are involved in walking and running, maintaining muscle tone and posture, sneezing, coughing, and breathing.

WHAT IS NERVE GAS?

Nerve gas is a term used for chemical warfare agents, such as sarin, that induce illness and death by their effects on neurotransmission. Most nerve agents are organophosphates—chemicals that were originally developed as and are still widely used as pesticides. First synthesized in 1854, widespread use of pesticides began in Germany in the 1920s. About 2,000 compounds (including tabun, sarin, and soman) were developed by German chemists as potential chemical warfare agents in the 1930s and 1940s but were never actually used in battle. Organophosphates, which are absorbed through the skin and the respiratory and digestive tracts, bind irreversibly to acetylcholinesterase, preventing the breakdown of acetylcholine in the synapse. Overstimulation of receptors in motor endplates causes muscle spasms, convulsions, and eventually paralysis of the muscles, including the diaphragm. Contractions of smooth muscle in the urinary tract, digestive tract, and secretory glands cause the group of cholinergic symptoms referred to as "SLUDGE": salivation, lacrimation (tear secretion), urination, diaphoresis (sweating), gastrointestinal distress (including diarrhea), and emesis (vomiting). Heart rate and respiration are also affected. Early treatment with anticholinergic drugs (such as atropine) that block cholinergic receptors and oximes (such as praloxidime) that break the bond of the nerve agent with acetylcholinesterase will avert death. Continued widespread use of organophosphates as pesticides has resulted in over 1 million cases of poisoning and 20,000 deaths per year worldwide, with the primary cause of injury and mortality being respiratory failure.

Basal Ganglia

Located at the base of the cerebral hemispheres, the basal ganglia in each hemisphere consist of the **caudate nucleus**, the **putamen**, the **nucleus accumbens**, the **globus pallidus**, and the **subthalamic nucleus** (Figure 5.3). Also included in the basal ganglia is a midbrain structure called the **substantia nigra**. If any of these nuclei are damaged, the person will experience severe movement problems. Among the many interconnections between the basal ganglia, and between the basal ganglia and the thalamus and cortex, scientists have found what they refer to as four anatomical "loops." The skeletomotor loop is involved with learned movements. In this loop, information from the primary motor and primary somatosensory cortices travels to the putamen. The putamen then sends the information to the globus pallidus, which projects to the ventrolateral and ventral anterior thalamic nuclei. These structures complete the loop by projecting back to the primary and premotor cortices. The prefrontal cortex loop plays a part in the conscious planning of movements. It begins when the caudate nucleus receives information from all **association areas** (secondary and higher-order sensory areas) of the cortex. The caudate nucleus projects to the globus pallidus, which then projects to the ventral anterior thalamic nucleus. This nucleus then completes the loop by projecting to the prefrontal cortex. Information in the limbic loop travels from the amygdala and cingulate gyrus (both part of the limbic system), going first to the nucleus accumbens and from there to the globus pallidus. The globus pallidus projects to the **dorsomedial thalamic nucleus**, which in turn projects to the supplementary motor cortex and the premotor cortex. Finally, the **oculomotor loop** participates in the control of eye movements. It begins in control centers for eye movement in the frontal lobe and in higher order visual cortex in the posterior parietal lobe. It travels from these areas to the substantia nigra, then to the ventral anterior thalamic nucleus,

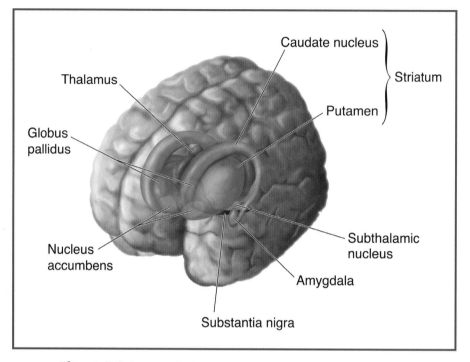

Figure 5.3 Input to the basal ganglia is received by the striatum. After incoming information is processed, the output nuclei— the ventral pallidum, the substantia nigra pars reticulata, and the globus pallidus internal segment—project to thalamic nuclei, the pedunculopontine nucleus, and the superior colliculus. These output pathways control movements of the limb, trunk, eye, and facial muscles. Other basal ganglia nuclei—the subthalamic nucleus and the external segment of the globus pallidus—are part of an intrinsic basal ganglia pathway that inhibits movement production.

and finally back to the prefrontal cortex and higher-order visual areas of the frontal cortex.

Cerebellum

The cerebral cortex has about 22 billion neurons. Even though it is smaller, the cerebellum actually has more neurons—about 50 billion. The cerebellum is connected to the brainstem by three pairs of cerebellar peduncles, or large bundles of fibers. Like the cerebrum, the cerebellum has two hemispheres, which are joined by a small structure called the **vermis**. The cerebellum has deep fissures that divide it into three horizontal lobes: an anterior lobe, a middle lobe, and a flocculonodular lobe.

Although scientists are not yet sure about all of the cerebellum's functions, they believe it coordinates all voluntary and reflex movements and helps us maintain proper muscle tone and normal body posture. When someone has an injury to the cerebellum, he or she may have trouble walking in a straight line or standing still without falling over—much like a person who has had too much alcohol to drink. In fact, it is the cerebellum that is impaired by excess alcohol intake. The cerebellum receives signals about voluntary movements from the cerebral cortex and, by way of the spinal cord, from the tendons, muscles, and joints. Input from the vestibular nerve also provides information relating to balance. The cerebellum helps the body coordinate fine and complex movements. It is involved, for example, in allowing you to pat your head and rub your stomach at the same time. The cerebellum is also involved in motor learning, and recent research indicates that it may play a role in higher cognitive functions as well as emotional and autonomic nervous system functions.

Motor Neurons

Eye muscles, facial muscles, and muscles that control tongue, jaw, and swallowing movements are innervated by neurons found in the motor nuclei of cranial nerves. Cranial nerves exit the brainstem and travel through openings in the skull to reach their targets. The vagus nerve, which is the longest cranial nerve, travels down the neck to reach the body cavity. There, it innervates viscera of the chest and abdomen as well as the large blood vessels of the chest.

Motor neurons are located in the ventral, or anterior, "wings" of the spinal cord gray matter. The spinal cord has two types of motor neurons: alpha motor neurons and gamma motor neurons. **Alpha motor neurons** send commands that make muscles contract. **Gamma motor neurons** are smaller than

TOXINS THAT AFFECT THE MOTOR NEURONS

Alpha motor neurons send collateral axons to interneurons called **Renshaw cells**. Renshaw cells send back an inhibitory signal, which helps the motor neurons to self-regulate. The neurotransmitter used by the Renshaw cell is the inhibitory neurotransmitter glycine. The bacterium *Clostridium tetani* releases tetanus toxin. This poison prevents the release of glycine from the presynaptic terminal of the Renshaw cell. Similarly, the poison strychnine blocks glycine receptors in the postsynaptic membrane of the alpha motor neuron. Both toxins prevent the Renshaw cells from inhibiting the alpha motor neurons, which results in convulsions. Because there are a large number of glycine receptors in the cranial nerve nuclei which innervate the facial expression muscles and jaw muscles, these two toxins particularly affect these two groups of muscles. "Lockjaw," the common name for tetanus, describes one of the symptoms of poisoning with the tetanus toxin: The teeth become clenched because of severe contractions of the jaw muscles.

In contrast, the botulinum toxin prevents the release of acetylcholine. This toxin is released by *Clostridium botulinum* and causes botulism, a type of food poisoning. Preventing the release of acetylcholine makes it impossible for the motor neurons and the preganglionic neurons to send signals to the muscles and internal organs. The result is that the muscles of movement, the muscles of the eyelid and pupil, and the muscles of the diaphragm, urinary bladder, bowel, and salivary glands become paralyzed. People suffering from this condition often have drooping eyelids, double vision, weak limb and facial muscles, and ultimately, paralysis of the respiratory muscles, which makes them unable to breathe on their own.

alpha motor neurons. They send signals that make muscle spindles more sensitive to external stimuli under certain conditions.

Motor neurons and interneurons are found in the spinal cord's gray matter. They are arranged in clusters that activate individual muscles. Those that innervate the neck and trunk muscles are located close to the midline in the ventral gray matter beneath the spinal canal. Upper and lower limbs are innervated by motor neurons that are in the lateral gray matter of the ventral spinal cord. In general, the farther the limb muscles are from the trunk, the more lateral the neurons that innervate them are located in the ventral gray matter.

REFLEXES

Spinal reflexes are involuntary movements that occur in response to sensory stimuli. These movements involve a circuit from one or more muscles to the spinal cord and back. The simplest reflexes involve just one motor neuron. These are referred to as monosynaptic reflexes. Other reflexes, called polysynaptic reflexes, involve two or more synapses, at least one of which involves an interneuron. Most reflexes are polysynaptic.

The only known example of the monosynaptic reflex is the stretch reflex. If a muscle fiber is stretched, a signal goes from the muscle spindle through a proprioreceptive fiber that synapses on the alpha motor neuron in the spinal cord. The alpha motor neuron responds by firing more often, which strengthens the contraction of the muscle fiber. An example of this is the knee jerk, or patellar reflex. When a doctor taps the patellar tendon beneath your knee with a small hammer, your thigh muscle stretches. This makes the muscle spindles fire and contract the thigh muscle, causing your lower leg to kick upward. When we lift a heavy object, the muscles in our arm increase their contractions in response to stretch, giving us the strength we need to support the weight. The stretching of the calf muscle that occurs when we lean forward makes it contract, which allows us to maintain an upright posture.

Withdrawal reflexes, also known as flexor reflexes, allow us to immediately remove a part of our body from a painful stimulus by flexing the limb involved. The brainstem normally sends out signals that keep the reflex pathways somewhat inhibited. Only painful or noxious stimuli cause us to have a strong reflexive action. Fibers from sensory neurons in the skin synapse on interneurons in the spinal cord, which, in turn, synapse on alpha motor neurons that synapse on and activate flexor muscles that move the limb away from the danger. Normally, the limb flexes to withdraw from the stimulus, but sometimes the brain has to activate the extensor muscles of another limb to withdraw it safely. A crossed extensor reflex involves the inhibition or activation (whichever is opposite) of the alpha motor neurons to the same muscle or group of muscles on the opposite side of the body. This allows you to alternate muscle movements during locomotion and helps maintain your posture during a withdrawal reflex. The brain can also send out signals to inhibitory neurons to override the withdrawal reflex. Sometimes this is necessary—for example, when you need to avoid dropping a hot object you are carrying.

CONNECTIONS

About 1 million motor neurons in the spinal cord control the movements of our arm, leg, foot, hand, and trunk muscles. Neurons in cranial nerve motor nuclei perform a similar function for muscles in the head, neck, face, and eyes. Spinal and cranial nerve motor neurons are under the direct influence of neurons in the cerebral cortex and brainstem and the indirect influence of neurons in the cerebellum. Fiber pathways descend from the cerebral cortex to cranial nerve nuclei and the spinal cord. The cerebellum influences the information that goes through these pathways by sending projections to the cerebral cortex and the brainstem nuclei involved. Somatosensory information relayed from the body via the spinal cord, as well as information that comes from the cerebral cortex and the brainstem, are processed by the cerebellum and influence its outputs. Located at the base of each cerebral hemisphere, the basal ganglia nuclei have complex interconnections with each other and with the thalamus and the cerebral cortex. Some of these interconnections are involved in learning and planning movements. Others allow control of the eye movements and the involvement of drives and emotions in motor responses.

6

Learning and Memory

From the time we take our first breath (and probably even before), we are continually learning. We learn to walk, run, ride a bicycle, read, write, interact with our environments, and much, much more. At the same time, we form memories that help us relate newly learned information to things we have learned previously.

TYPES OF LEARNING

There are four basic types of learning: perceptual, stimulus-response, motor, and relational. One or more of these types is active in any given learning situation.

Perceptual Learning

Perceptual learning allows us to recognize and identify stimuli we have encountered before. Changes in the higher-order cortex, or association cortex, that are associated with each of the senses allow us to recognize these stimuli when we encounter them again. Scientists believe that memories for each sensory modality are stored in a specific sensory association cortex.

Stimulus-Response Learning

Stimulus-response learning includes **classical conditioning** and **instrumental conditioning**. These occur when we learn to respond in a certain way to a particular stimulus. The response can be as simple as a defensive reflex or as complicated as a sequence of movements. Classical conditioning or **associative learning**, takes place when we learn to associate a previously neutral stimulus with one that naturally produces a reflexive response. Eventually, we respond to the "neutral" stimulus even when the stimulus that was originally responsible for the reflex is no longer there. This type of conditioning was discovered by Russian physiologist, Ivan Pavlov, who was studying salivation in dogs as part of his Nobel Prize–winning research on digestion. He discovered that the dogs he was using for research would salivate at the sight of food or even at his appearance in the room. Through experimentation, he learned that if he rang a bell each time before he fed the dogs, they would eventually learn to salivate in response to the bell, even in the absence of food.

Instrumental conditioning is a type of learning that occurs when we learn to associate either a reinforcer or a punisher with a particular response or behavior. This is the type of learning that occurs in a Skinner box when a rat learns to press a lever for food or to avoid a negative stimulus such as an electrical shock. The Skinner box was invented by American psychologist B. F. Skinner. Skinner used the box extensively to explore the principles of instrumental conditioning. He found out, for example, that varying the number of times a rat had to press a lever to get a food pellet would affect the rate at which the rat pressed the lever. Skinner believed, correctly, that instrumental conditioning, also called operant learning, would work with people as well. People, too, will increase behaviors for which they receive positive consequences and decrease behaviors for which they receive negative consequences. Skinner invented programmed instruction, in which the learner gets step-by-step feedback on the material he or she is learning.

Motor Learning

Motor learning is the learning of skilled movements, such as knitting, typing, playing a piano, riding a bicycle, or dancing. Although we make these movements slowly and deliberately when we first learn them, they become automatic after we've had a lot of practice. As we will learn later, motor learning involves a shifting of control of the learned movements from a conscious type of memory system to an unconscious type of memory system.

Relational Learning

Relational learning involves learning relationships between multiple stimuli. It results in the formation of neural connections between the various areas of higher order sensory cortex involved. Examples of relational learning include more complex forms of perceptual learning, spatial learning, episodic learning, and observational learning. Perceptual learning that involves more than one sensory modality requires the formation of connections between the sensory association cortices involved. **Spatial learning** involves learning about the objects in the surrounding environment and their locations with respect to each other and to the learner. **Episodic learning** involves remembering events and the order, or sequence, in which they occur. **Observational learning** occurs when we learn by observing and imitating the actions of other people. In this type of learning, relationships between actions, consequences, and one's own movements must be learned.

PHASES OF MEMORY FORMATION

Learning is often defined as the process of acquiring knowledge, with memory being the end result (Figure 6.1). There are three basic aspects of memory formation: encoding, storage, and retrieval. **Encoding** is the process by which stimuli from the environment are changed into a neural code that can be perceived by the brain. **Storage**, or **consolidation**, is the process by which this encoded information is recorded in memory. **Retrieval** is the process by which information is accessed in the memory stores. Information stored in memory may be retrieved by conscious recall of specific information or by recognition of previously encountered information, such as a name, word, or place.

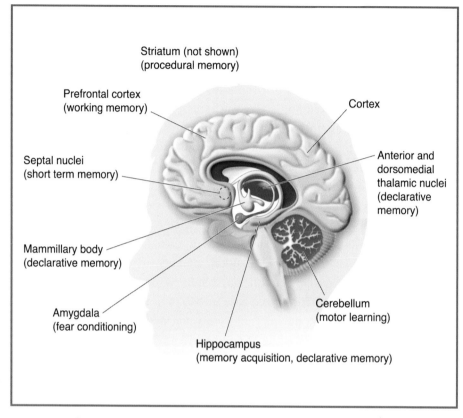

Figure 6.1 The structures that have been most strongly implicated in memory functions are shown here. Damage to these structures by disease or injury will produce a loss of memory. The memory loss of Alzheimer's disease is generally attributed to the significant damage to the hippocampus seen with that disease.

STAGES OF MEMORY

Before it is stored in the brain, information goes through three stages of processing. Most of the information we get from our environment never gets beyond the first stage—**sensory memory**. Sensory memory lasts only milliseconds or seconds at most. It includes all the stimuli that comes to us from the environment. If we focus on or pay attention to particular stimuli, that information will enter our

short-term memory (also known as **immediate memory** or working memory). This type of memory lasts from seconds to minutes and can store 7 (plus or minus 2) items. **Rehearsal**, or repetition, of the information in short-term memory helps us keep it there longer. If the information is important enough, it may then be transferred into **long-term memory** storage in the brain, where it can remain for a lifetime. Long-term memory has an enormous capacity. It includes all the facts and knowledge that we accumulate throughout our entire lives—from the rules of English grammar to the lyrics of your favorite song.

Long-term memory includes two major classes: explicit memory and implicit memory, which, in turn, have subclasses of their own (Figure 6.2). **Explicit memory**, or **declarative memory**, is available to the conscious mind and can be declared, or put into words. There are two subclasses of explicit memory: episodic memory and semantic memory. **Episodic memory** is the recollection of past experiences, or episodes, in our lives. These memories might be as recent as what you ate for breakfast today or as far back as your first day at elementary school. **Semantic memory** stores information that is not related to a particular experience. Instead, it includes such things as word meanings, ideas, and facts. Most of the factual knowledge we gain in the classroom or from reading books is stored as semantic memory.

Implicit memory, or **nondeclarative memory**, is stored information that is not available to conscious thought. It cannot be put into words easily. Subclasses of implicit memory include memories that result from classical conditioning, memories that make priming possible, and procedural memory. Priming occurs when a cue such as a card containing the first three letters of a word helps us retrieve information stored in unconscious memory. **Procedural memory** includes rules that we learn unconsciously (without realizing it) and memories that result from motor learning. Examples of procedural

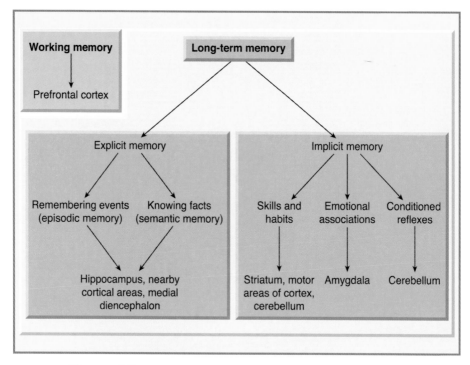

Figure 6.2 The most commonly described types of memory are depicted here with the anatomical structures with which they have been associated through research. Some of these correlations are still speculative, particularly those involving the striatum and cerebellum.

memory include learning rules of grammar or learning how to play a musical instrument.

ANATOMY OF LEARNING AND MEMORY
The Limbic System

A group of structures called the limbic system works together to produce and regulate our emotions and to form new memories (Figure 6.3). There are two subsystems of the limbic system—one in which the hippocampus plays a central role, and the other in which the amygdala is the key structure. Since the amygdala plays a key role in the regulation of emotions, we will discuss

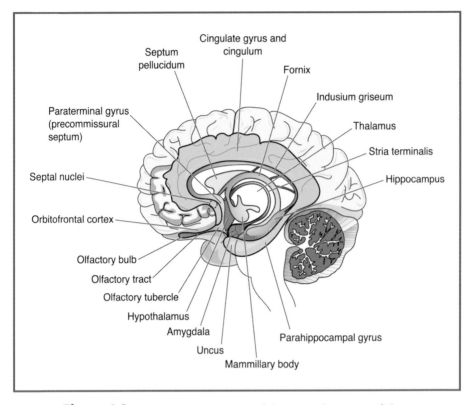

Figure 6.3 The major components of the two subsystems of the limbic system, which center around the hippocampus and the amygdala, are shown here. Subcortical components shown include the hippocampus, amygdala, hypothalamus, thalamus, and olfactory tubercle. Cortical components include the cingulate gyrus, the parahippocampal gyrus, and the orbitofrontal cortex. Also shown is the induseum griseum, or hippocampal rudiment, which is continuous with the hippocampus and represents the descent of the hippocampus from above the lateral ventricles to the medial temporal lobe during embryological development.

the second subsystem in Chapter 7. Although it performs other functions also, the hippocampus is necessary for acquiring new memories. Scientists believe that the hippocampus is the structure where explicit memory is consolidated before it is transferred to the cerebral cortex for long-term storage.

Surrounding the diencephalon at the base of the brain is a horseshoe-shaped area of cortex that includes the cingulate gyri and the parahippocampal gyri, which are part of the limbic association cortex. The cingulum is a fiber bundle that runs beneath the surface of the cingulate gyrus and brings information from the sensory and other association areas in the cortex to the parahippocampal gyrus, which is the cortex that overlies the hippocampus. The entorhinal cortex, which is the rostral, or front part, of the parahippocampal gyrus, relays to the hippocampus the information that the cingulum brings in. It also relays information to the hippocampus that it receives from the orbital cortex, another limbic association cortex, the olfactory tract, and the amygdala.

The hippocampus receives direct projections from the septal nuclei and the hypothalamus through a large fiber bundle called the **fornix** and information through the **hippocampal commissure**. Direct projections to the hippocampus also come from the raphe nuclei, the locus coeruleus, and the ventral striatum. The hippocampus sends information back to the entorhinal cortex, which then sends widespread projections to the cortex. The fornix carries information from the hippocampus to the mammillary bodies and the septal nuclei.

The Hippocampus

Anatomically, the **hippocampal formation** is made up of the **dentate gyrus**, the **hippocampus proper**, and the **subiculum**. Damage to the hippocampus or its input or output regions and fibers results in memory loss, or amnesia. Hippocampal damage can result from head trauma, aneurysms (saclike protrusions from a blood vessel that form because the vessel wall weakens) of arteries that supply the hippocampus, epileptic seizures, or loss of oxygen supply (hypoxia) during cardiac arrest. One of the first structures to show damage during aging or as a result of Alzheimer's disease is the hippocampus.

Damage to both hippocampi results in **anterograde amnesia**, or the inability to learn new information. **Retrograde amnesia**, the loss of previously learned information, may be present as well. Loss of memory for events that occurred from 1 year up to as many as 15 years before the damage may be present in some individuals. The most famous example of anterograde amnesia is the case of a patient known to science as "H. M." In an attempt to stop his epileptic seizures, about two inches of H. M.'s medial temporal lobe, including the amygdala, about two-thirds of the hippocampus, and the overlying cortex, were surgically removed on each side (Figure 6.4). Ever since the operation, which occurred in 1953, scientists have studied H. M. continuously. Although he can store new information temporarily in his short-term memory, he can no longer form any new long-term memories. Rehearsal of information in his short-term memory allows him to hold on to information until he is distracted, at which point he loses the memory. In contrast to his inability to form new memories, H. M.'s retrograde memory loss is limited to a period of 11 years prior to his surgery at age 27. His memories formed before age 16 are still intact. Although H. M. learns and retains motor skills, he cannot remember having learned them or having performed them.

Studies in animals and in human patients like H. M. have shown that damage to the hippocampus causes problems in explicit memory but not in implicit memory. (Explicit memory is information to which our conscious mind has access. Implicit memory cannot be deliberately recalled.) This suggests that there may be multiple memory systems within the brain. Free recall of information, as well as recognition memory, the ability to recall previously encountered information, is impaired after hippocampal damage. Neuroimaging studies that use memory tasks in humans have shown that the hippocampus is active during both the formation and retrieval of memories.

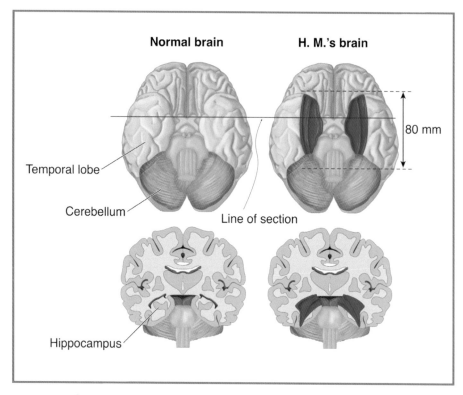

Figure 6.4 In the upper right figure, the areas of the medial temporal lobe that were removed on both sides of H. M.'s brain are shown. This view is of the ventral surface, or undersurface, of the brain. The horizontal line across the two upper figures shows where the brain would be cut to produce the sections shown in the two lower figures. In the lower right figure, you can see that the hippocampus and overlying cortex are missing. The two figures on the left show a normal brain for comparison.

Midline Diencephalic Nuclei

Damage to diencephalic structures adjacent to the third ventricle, such as the midthalamic nuclei and the mammillary bodies, also causes amnesia. Korsakoff's syndrome, which is usually caused by severe thiamine deficiency resulting from years of alcohol abuse, results in damage to the mammillary bodies and other structures. One of the symptoms of Korsakoff's syndrome is anterograde amnesia. Strokes that affect the thalamus can also cause amnesia. Amnesia resulting from damage to these diencephalic structures probably occurs because of their connections to other structures, such as the hippocampus and the frontal cortex.

Prefrontal Cortex

Areas in the frontal cortex appear to be involved in planning, problem solving, and in the organizational strategies used in memory tasks. Results of neuroimaging studies have suggested that the left inferior (lower) prefrontal cortex is important in encoding information for storage and in conceptual processing, or processing related to the meaning of words. Other neuroimaging studies have shown that an area of the right prefrontal cortex is involved in retrieving memories. Studies of patients with frontal lobe damage and neuroimaging studies of frontal lobe activity have shown that the frontal lobes are involved in holding onto the information we need for ongoing tasks in short-term or working memory. There is increased activation of the prefrontal cortex during working memory tasks, such as remembering a phone number long enough to dial it.

The Basal Ganglia and Cerebellum

Research suggests that once the skills we learn become automatic (when we can perform them without thinking about them consciously), control of these behaviors moves from the basal ganglia to the sensory and motor association cortices. The caudate and putamen nuclei get information about movements from the frontal cortex. They also receive sensory information from all cortical regions. As the outputs of the caudate and putamen nuclei go to the globus pallidus, which sends the information to the primary, premotor, and supplementary motor cortices, a loop is formed. Projections from the globus pallidus also travel to the dorsomedial thalamic nucleus, which projects to cognitive areas of the frontal lobe.

Laboratory animals with damage to the basal ganglia have problems with instrumental conditioning. People who suffer from Huntington's disease or Parkinson's disease, who have degenerative damage to their basal ganglia, experience both cognitive and motor problems. Patients with Parkinson's disease show slowness of thought, have a hard time switching from one task to another, and find it difficult to interpret nonverbal social cues ("body language"). Patients with Huntington's disease have even more severe cognitive impairment and frequently suffer from dementia.

Another loop goes from the motor cortex to the cerebellum and back to the cortex by way of the thalamus. This loop appears to play a role in motor skill learning. Activity in both loops has been observed in neuroimaging studies of motor learning. The cerebellum seems to be most involved when we first perform a motor learning task. As we practice the task, the cerebellum's involvement decreases. By the time the practiced skill becomes automatic, the involvement of the cerebellum can no longer be detected. However, basal ganglia involvement appears to be greatest after the skill becomes automatic and does not decrease after that point.

Motor Association Cortex

Given the involvement of the premotor and supplementary cortices in motor planning and the fact that they are the target of most of the information relayed from the basal ganglia through the thalamus, it would be reasonable to assume that the motor association cortex is involved in motor learning. Research has shown that damage to the supplementary motor cortex impairs self-initiated movements and the performance of a sequence of movements. A positron emission tomography, or PET (neuroimaging), study in humans backed up this observation by demonstrating that the supplementary motor cortex is activated during learning and in the performance of a sequence of movements. Some scientists believe that memories are stored in the sensory association cortices associated with the different senses and in the areas involved in the performance of a particular task. If these scientists are correct, then the motor association cortex, along with the cerebellum and the basal ganglia, would be some of the places where motor learning information is most likely to be stored.

The Amygdala

Memory consolidation is enhanced by epinephrine (adrenaline) and glucocorticoids (cortisol), which are stress hormones released by the adrenal glands. Research indicates that stress hormones cause the amygdala's basolateral nucleus to release norepinephrine. (Epinephrine also causes the liver to release glucose, the primary fuel of the brain.) Footshock and certain drugs that enhance the consolidation of memory also increase the release of norepinephrine in the basolateral nucleus. Activation of cholinergic muscarinic receptors in the basolateral amygdala appears to be important for the effects of glucocorticoids on memory consolidation enhancement. Some scientists think the amygdala may be the site where the neural changes that produce learned fear occur. But most research indicates that the role of the amygdala in memory consolidation is a modulatory one that affects other brain areas.

PHYSIOLOGY OF LEARNING AND MEMORY

Learning and memory processes produce synaptic changes in the neural circuits that they activate. Studies have shown that the brains of rats raised in an enriched environment—where they had access to other rats, slides, ladders, running wheels, and toys—weighed more and had a thicker cortex, more glial cells, a better blood supply, and larger postsynaptic areas than rats raised alone in a cage with no external stimulation. In one study, rats that were exposed to the extensive visual stimulation of training in a maze had larger dendritic trees on the neurons in their visual cortex.

CONNECTIONS

Learning allows us to recognize stimuli in our environment and their relationships to each other, and to respond to them appropriately. It also helps us develop skilled behaviors that let us interact with our environment. Learned information is stored in memory so we can use it in the future. Important stimuli from the environment are encoded from immediate memory into short-term memory, which has limited storage capacity. Information that is important enough or has been rehearsed can be put into long-term memory, which has a very large storage capacity. Explicit memory, but not implicit memory, is accessible to conscious thought processes. Semantic

COGNITIVE REHABILITATION THERAPY

Cognitive rehabilitation therapy is designed to restore or compensate for cognitive functions lost due to stroke, trauma, disease, tumor, or deficits in brain development. A neuropsychologist, physical therapist, or speech therapist usually conducts this type of therapy. Vision therapists also offer treatment for visual memory and visual perception problems. A number of computer programs have been designed for use both in the therapist's office and at home. The activities and computer programs improve or strengthen memory, visual perception, attention, learning skills, cognitive processing speed, problem solving and reasoning, abstract and critical thinking, and impulse control.

Feuerstein's Instrumental Enrichment program is a related type of therapy that emphasizes the idea of "cognitive modifiability." This concept suggests that intelligence is not fixed; instead, it can be modified. Thinking skills are taught with a series of tasks that gradually become more complex and abstract. This program has not only been used clinically but is also being used in classrooms to help students "learn how to learn."

and episodic memory—remembering facts and events, respectively—are forms of explicit memory. Memories that form through conditioning and motor learning, as well as the learning of rules, are examples of implicit memory. Structures of the limbic system, particularly the hippocampus, are believed to be involved in the processes that underlie learning and memory. Areas in the prefrontal cortex also appear to be involved in helping the brain organize memory tasks, encoding and retrieving information, and holding information in working memory. Basal ganglia structures and the cerebellum are important for motor skill learning and possibly other cognitive functions. Emotional memories may be consolidated in the amygdala.

7

Emotions and Reward Systems

You might say that emotions add the "flavor" to life's activities and the "color" to our memories. Depending on the situation, they can lift us to the heights of exhilaration or plunge us into the depths of despair. Most of our emotions, however, lie somewhere between these two extremes. What most of us do not realize is that the feelings that accompany these emotions are powered by physiological changes that are put into motion by the central nervous system. In this chapter, we will take a look at the brain structures involved in both positive and negative emotions and the neural connections that allow the integration of the psychological and physiological components of emotion.

NEUROANATOMY OF EMOTIONS

Just as the hippocampus is the central structure in memory formation, the amygdala is the major structure in the creation and expression of emotions. Like the hippocampus, the amygdala has both direct and indirect interconnections with the cerebral cortex. Both the amygdala and the hippocampus also have direct connections to the hypothalamus and indirect connections to the thalamus.

The Amygdala

Scientists disagree on how many groups to place the nuclei of the amygdala in. Some say two (basolateral and corticomedial), some say three (basolateral, central, and corticomedial), and some say four, as shown in Figure 7.1. Research has shown that the basolateral nuclei function to give a stimulus emotional significance. Sensory information goes to the basolateral amygdala from the secondary and higher-order sensory cortices from all areas of the cortex. After processing this information, the basolateral amygdala sends both direct and indirect projections to the cortex.

The emotional response consists of both physiological (autonomic and hormonal) and behavioral components. It is regulated by the central nuclei, which play a role in the control of the autonomic nervous system. Sensory information from the cortex is relayed through the basolateral nuclei to the central nuclei. Emotional learning associated with **aversive stimuli** is also modulated by the central nuclei, which studies have shown is necessary for the conditioned emotional response task (CER). CER is a learning task in which animals exhibit fear after being trained to associate a tone or other stimulus with an aversive stimulus such as an electrical shock. Output from the central nuclei to the lateral hypothalamus leads to the characteristic physiological response to fear: increased blood pressure, activation of the sympathetic nervous system, and the production of stress hormones by the adrenal glands. The central nuclei, as well as the basolateral nuclei, are also important in addiction and substance abuse. The amygdala also sends fibers to the sympathetic preganglionic neurons in the spinal cord.

There are also inputs from the hypothalamus and central nuclei to the midbrain **periaqueductal gray area**, which surrounds the cerebral aqueduct and mediates species-specific motor responses, such as hissing and growling, to emotional stimuli. Secretion of corticotropin releasing hormone (CRH) from the hypothalamic paraventricular nucleus, the first step in a pathway that ends with the secretion of cortisol from the adrenal medulla, is increased by disinhibition produced by projections from the central nuclei of the amygdala. Positive

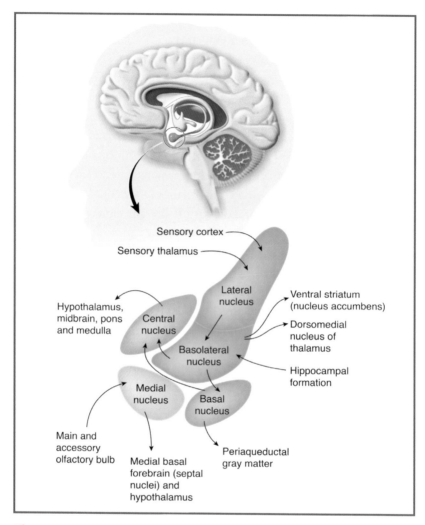

Figure 7.1 Some scientists divide the nuclei of the amygdala into four groups as shown here. The lateral/basolateral nuclei have direct reciprocal connections with higher-order sensory cortices and the hippocampus and also send relays to the cortex through the thalamus and basal forebrain. Sensory information received by the basal nuclei from the lateral/basolateral nuclei is relayed to the periaqueductal gray matter and to other amygdaloid nuclei. The central nuclei receive information from the lateral/basolateral nuclei and from the brainstem and project to the lateral hypothalamus and the brainstem to regulate the autonomic nervous system. Medial nuclei receive primary olfactory information and relay it to the hypothalamus and medial basal forebrain.

feedback through fibers from the CRH neurons to the central nuclei increases CRH secretion further.

The basolateral amygdala is also part of the basal ganglia limbic loop, which begins in the ventral striatum (nucleus accumbens), an area that has direct reciprocal connections with the amygdala. Information from the hippocampus, the limbic association cortex, and all four divisions of the amygdala arrives in the ventral striatum, which processes this information and sends its output to the ventral globus pallidus. After relaying in the medial dorsal nucleus of the thalamus, the ventral pallidal output reaches the prefrontal cortex, the anterior cingulate gyrus, and the medial orbitofrontal cortex. These areas then project to the premotor cortex, which, in turn, projects to the primary motor cortex for the execution of movements.

There are two major output pathways from the amygdala: the **stria terminalis** and the **amygdalofugal pathway**. Most of the fibers in the stria terminalis go to and from the cortico-medial nuclei. In its descent to the hypothalamic ventromedial nucleus (its primary target), the stria terminalis follows a C-shaped path along the caudate nucleus and lateral ventricle. Fibers also pass from one amygdala to the other through the stria terminalis and then across the **anterior commissure**. The **bed nucleus of the stria terminalis** follows the course of the fiber pathway and has projections and functions similar to those of the central nuclei. Most of the fibers that course through the amygdalofugal pathway go to and from the basolateral and central nuclear divisions. There are also fibers that connect the amygdalar nuclei to other structures without passing through these two major fiber pathways.

Like other major structures of the limbic system, the amygdala receives projections from dopaminergic, seroto-nergic, and adrenergic nuclei in the brainstem as well as the cholinergic septal nuclei through the **median forebrain bundle**. This is an important fiber pathway through which fibers from each of these neurotransmitter systems travel.

The Frontal Lobes

Although the amygdala is important in evaluating emotional significance and generating involuntary behavioral, autonomic, and neuroendocrine responses to stimuli, the frontal lobes are involved in the conscious experience of emotions and in controlling emotional behavior. Located on the underside of each cerebral hemisphere (just above the bones of the eye sockets), the **orbitofrontal cortex** is the area that appears to be most directly involved in emotions.

In a surgical procedure known as **prefrontal lobotomy**, the fiber pathways to and from the frontal lobes, mainly those to and from the orbitofrontal cortex, are disconnected from the rest of the brain to relieve emotional distress. Egas Moniz, the Portuguese neuropsychiatrist who introduced the procedure in the late 1930s, received a Nobel Prize for Physiology or

THE STRANGE STORY OF PHINEAS GAGE

An unusual case illustrates very clearly just how important the frontal lobes are. In 1848, a 25-year-old construction worker named Phineas Gage was injured in an explosion while on the job. A 3-foot-long metal rod shot up through Gage's skull. Miraculously, he survived. However, the people who knew him quickly noticed some major changes in his personality. Before the accident, Gage had been friendly and hardworking. After the injury to the frontal lobes of his brain, though, he suddenly became ornery, loud, and unstable in his moods. Scientists today know that the area of Gage's brain that was damaged—the prefrontal cortex—is responsible for regulating emotions. Because this part of his brain could no longer function, Gage had no real control over his feelings and impulses. Gage was left unable to return to his construction job. After the accident, he primarily worked in livery stables and drove coaches, and also made an appearance at P. T. Barnum's museum in New York.

Medicine in 1949 for developing this procedure. In some of the surgeries performed as the procedure became popular, the ventral connections of the frontal lobes with the temporal lobes and diencephalon were cut. In others, dorsal connections were severed between the frontal lobes and the cingulate gyrus. Unfortunately, the procedure eliminated both pathological reactions *and* normal emotional reactions. Though intellectual ability was not harmed by the operation, patients developed severe personality changes. They often became childish and irresponsible, were unable to carry out plans, and were usually left unemployable. Thousands of these surgeries were done before the procedure was finally abandoned because of its harmful side effects.

REWARD MECHANISMS

Natural reinforcers (such as food, water, and sex) stimulate the "pleasure centers" of the brain. So, too, do addictive drugs—including cocaine, amphetamines, cannabis, heroin, morphine, alcohol, nicotine, and caffeine. These natural and artificial reinforcers increase the release of the neurotransmitter dopamine in the nucleus accumbens. The nucleus accumbens is the site where the caudate and putamen nuclei fuse. It is sometimes referred to as the ventral striatum. The dopamine released in the nucleus accumbens is synthesized by dopaminergic neurons that project to the nucleus accumbens from the ventral tegmental area (VTA).

There are a number of "pleasure centers" in the brain for which rats will press a lever to receive electrical stimulation through an electrode implanted there. Rats will press longest and hardest for stimulation of the median forebrain bundle, especially where it crosses the lateral hypothalamus. A rat will press the lever at a high rate for hours and neglect to eat or drink, preferring instead to obtain electrical stimulation through the electrode planted there. In the median forebrain bundle are found serotonergic and adrenergic fibers in

ALBERT AND THE WHITE RAT: CONDITIONED EMOTIONAL RESPONSE

A conditioned emotional response is actually a learned response in which a previously neutral stimulus becomes associated with a stimulus that naturally produces a pleasant or an unpleasant emotion. The most famous (or notorious) example can be found in the results of a series of experiments published by John B. Watson and his graduate student, Rosalie Rayner, in 1920. The study is often referred to as "Albert and the White Rat." Albert, a placid 9-month-old boy, was shown several items, including a white rat, a dog, a rabbit, a monkey, burning newspapers, and masks (some with hair). He did not react with fear to any of them. Subsequently, Watson and Rayner made a loud sound by striking a steel bar suspended behind Albert's head with a hammer. For the first time, Albert showed a fear response. Later, the researchers brought out the white rat again, and struck the bar with the hammer as Albert reached for the rat. Albert gradually became conditioned to fear the white rat and the other animals from the series of experiments that followed. His fear conditioning was still apparent at the age of one year, when Albert was tested with a Santa Claus mask, fur coat, white rat, rabbit, and dog. Unfortunately, the researchers lost contact with Albert, and never got the chance to extinguish his fear of the items. One of the conclusions that Watson and Rayner drew from this experiment was that phobias may be the result of fear conditioning that takes place at some point in one's life.

Scientists today continue to use the conditioned emotional response in animal research, typically in cases where a stimulus, such as a tone, is paired a number of times with a brief footshock and then alone during testing the following day. The physiological and behavioral responses elicited by the footshock alone before conditioning are elicited by the tone alone after conditioning. Of course, pleasant emotions can be and are paired with various stimuli during our daily lives, and many associations—both pleasant and unpleasant—some of them without our conscious awareness, strongly influence our behavior.

addition to the dopaminergic fibers. However, when the rats are given drugs that block dopaminergic receptors—but not when they are given those that block serotonergic or dopaminergic receptors—they reduce or even stop their lever-pressing for self-stimulation.

One characteristic that addictive drugs have in common is their ability to increase the release of dopamine in the nucleus accumbens. Cocaine increases the amount of dopamine, serotonin, and norepinephrine in a synapse by blocking their transporters from reuptaking them back into the presynaptic terminal. Amphetamines act to block reuptake and to increase the release of neurotransmitters. Caffeine stimulates dopamine release by blocking adenosine receptors, which inhibit dopamine release. Marijuana contains a substance called tetrahydrocannibol (THC) that binds to the cannaboid receptors, which are the sites where the endogenous (internally produced) cannaboids **anandamide** and **2-arachidonoyl** activate the VTA dopaminergic neurons. Binding to presynaptic nicotinic receptors, nicotine increases the excitatory effects of glutamatergic projections to the ventral tegmental area and decreases the inhibitory effects of GABAergic projections.

An increase in dopamine in the nucleus accumbens by reinforcers fulfills natural drives that promote health and well-being. Just as the amygdala is important in enhancing memories that are associated with negative stimuli, the nucleus accumbens helps reinforce memories associated with positive, or pleasurable, stimuli. Also like the amygdala, the nucleus accumbens acts as an interface between the emotional components of the limbic system and the behavioral-activating components of the motor system. Once positive or negative emotions have been associated with a stimulus, the prefrontal cortex chooses appropriate behavioral reactions, which the motor system carries out.

Addictive drugs cause the brain to release abnormally large amounts of dopamine. This leads to changes in the density

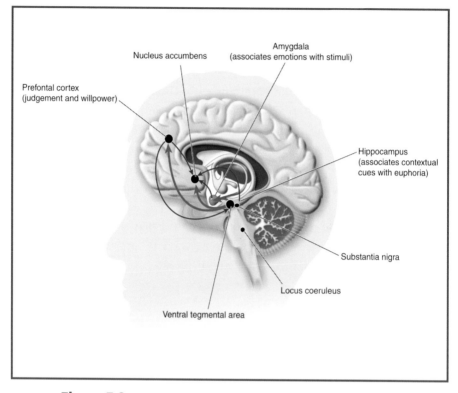

Figure 7.2 One action that drugs of abuse have in common is the stimulation of an increase in release of dopamine from neurons of the ventral tegmental area (VTA) that synapse in the nucleus accumbens. Some addictive drugs have actions in other brain structures as well. Depicted here are the basic dopaminergic pathways from the VTA to the nucleus accumbens, prefrontal cortex, and amygdala. Not shown is the indirect nondopaminergic pathway from the nucleus accumbens to the prefrontal cortex.

of dopaminergic receptors in the synapses, changes in other cellular mechanisms, and even changes in synaptic connections similar to those seen in learning and memory. When there is not enough of the drug in the body to fill the available receptors, the drug user experiences withdrawal symptoms. Some of the most common withdrawal symptoms include headaches, dizziness, irritability, and nervousness. In effect, in drug abuse, the body's natural reward system is taken over by the addictive drug so that it is driven to take more and more of the drug rather than to pursue potentially beneficial natural reinforcers (Figure 7.2).

The association of emotions with stimuli involves both its role in the control of learning and memory formation, which may explain why we recall emotional memories more easily and for longer than other memories. Some scientists believe there is a memory component of drug craving that is produced when the drug user associates the euphoria produced by the drug with the people, places, and paraphernalia that were present when the drug was taken. Drug addiction, therefore, may in some ways be considered a maladaptive form of learning and memory.

CONNECTIONS

Physiological components of emotional responses are regulated by the central amygdala through its control of the autonomic nervous system. Behavioral components of emotional responses are regulated through the involvement of the basolateral nucleus in the basal ganglia limbic loop and through projections from the central nucleus directly to the periaqueductal gray matter and indirectly to the reticular formation via the hypothalamus. The most important frontal lobe structure involved in emotions is the orbitofrontal cortex.

Reward, or pleasure, pathways in the brain involve the dopaminergic projections from the ventral tegmental area to the nucleus accumbens and the prefrontal cortex. Addictive drugs stimulate the release of dopamine in the nucleus accumbens. There appears to be a reward component and an associative learning component of addiction.

8

Neuroendocrine and Neuroimmune Interactions

THE HYPOTHALAMUS AND THE ENDOCRINE SYSTEM

The hypothalamus is the primary regulator of the endocrine system and autonomic nervous system—no small task for a structure that weighs only 4 grams, or 0.3% of the weight of the entire brain!

The hypothalamus controls the posterior lobe, or **neurohypophysis**, of the pituitary gland through neural output. Neurosecretory cells in the paraventricular and supraoptic nuclei of the hypothalamus produce the hormones vasopressin and oxytocin, which are released into the posterior lobe from axon terminals. (This means that, unlike the anterior pituitary, the posterior pituitary is actually part of the brain.) Once in the bloodstream, **vasopressin**, also known as **antidiuretic hormone** (**ADH**), helps regulate kidney function (Figure 8.1). It causes the kidney to reabsorb more water and decrease urine production. By causing the smooth muscle of blood vessels to contract, vasopressin also increases blood pressure. **Oxytocin** causes smooth muscles in the uterus and mammary glands to contract. Its action brings on the contractions of childbirth and the release of milk during breastfeeding. Table 8.1 lists some of the most important hormones of the hypothalamus and the effects they have on the body.

(continued on page 116)

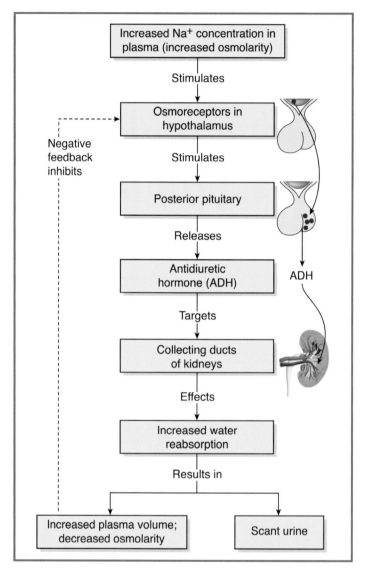

Figure 8.1 Antidiuretic hormone (ADH), also known as vasopressin, enters the bloodstream after being released in the posterior pituitary by axons from the hypothalamus. Drinking too much water will cause a decrease in the secretion of ADH. Dehydration will cause an increase in its secretion, making the kidneys retain more fluid. The process of ADH release and its effects on water retention and elimination are illustrated here.

Table 8.1 SOME IMPORTANT HYPOTHALAMIC HORMONES

HORMONE	SITE OF SYNTHESIS	FUNCTION
Corticotropin Releasing Hormone (CRH)	Paraventricular nucleus Arcuate nucleus Dorsomedial nucleus	Stimulates adrenocorticotropic releasing hormone (ACTH) production (triggers hypothalamic–pituito–adrenal axis)
Dopamine	Arcuate nucleus Periventricular nucleus	Inhibits thyroid stimulating hormone (TSH) and growth hormone (GH) release
Growth Hormone Releasing Hormone (GHRH)	Arcuate nucleus Perifornical area	Stimulates release of GH
Gonadotropin Releasing Hormone (GNRH)	Preoptic area Arcuate nucleus Periventricular nucleus Suprachiasmatic area	Stimulates release of gonadotropins* —follicle-stimulating hormone (FSH) and luteinizing hormone (LH)
Oxytocin	Paraventricular nucleus Supraoptic nucleus	Causes smooth muscle contraction for childbirth and milk ejection
Somatostatin	Arcuate nucleus Dorsomedial nucleus	Inhibits TSH and GH release
Thyrotropin Releasing Hormone (TRH)	Paraventricular nucleus (mostly) Perifornical area Suprachiasmatic nucleus	Stimulates release of TSH
Vasopressin	Paraventricular nucleus Supraoptic nucleus	Causes kidney to reabsorb more water; prevents dehydration

* FSH causes ovarian follicle development, and LH causes ovulation.

(continued from page 113)

The hypothalamus controls the release of hormones from the anterior lobe, or **adenohypophysis**, through its blood supply. Small peptides called hypothalamic releasing and inhibitory hormones are secreted from the axonal terminals of several hypothalamic nuclei into the stalk-like structure that connects the hypothalamus to the pituitary. These hormones enter the anterior pituitary through its extensive blood supply. Releasing hormones increase the production of pituitary hormones, and inhibiting hormones have the opposite effect.

The Hypothalamus and Homeostasis

Thermoreceptors in the hypothalamus detect changes in body temperature and send nerve signals to the autonomic nervous system. Activation of the autonomic nervous system produces the behavioral and physiological changes that are needed to adapt to the temperature of the environment.

Projections to the autonomic nervous system from the preoptic area and anterior hypothalamus produce increased sweating and **vasolidation** to let off heat. In animals, projections to the somatic motor system cause panting. Activation of the autonomic nervous system by the posterior hypothalamus causes shivering and vasoconstriction in the skin to produce and conserve heat.

Osmoreceptors in the hypothalamus detect changes in the concentration of certain substances such as sodium in the blood (blood **osmolarity**). Drinking too much water makes osmolarity decrease, whereas dehydration causes an increase in osmolarity. When osmolarity rises, it triggers a release of vasopressin. When osmolarity decreases, vasopressin secretion is reduced, which encourages the kidneys to excrete more water. Vasopressin secretion can also be activated by stress, pain, and certain emotional states.

The Hypothalamus and Ingestive Behavior

If the lateral area of the hypothalamus is damaged, food and water intake—and consequently, body weight—decreases. Within the lateral hypothalamus are neurons that contain orexin and melanin-concentrating hormone. These hormones influence feeding behavior. Eating (particularly of carbohydrates) is stimulated by the release of norepinephrine from the paraventricular nucleus, although it is not clear whether the eating behavior is a direct effect of the norepinephrine or an indirect effect of increased insulin secretion that occurs because of the intake of food. Galanin, a peptide that is also released with norepinephrine, stimulates us to eat more fats. Neuropeptide Y, which is synthesized in the arcuate nucleus, stimulates food intake by activating the "feeding center" in the lateral hypothalamus. Ghrelin, a peptide secreted by endocrine cells in the stomach lining, stimulates arcuate neurons, which also increases food intake.

Located in the ventromedial nucleus of the hypothalamus is a "**satiety** center." This part of the brain is activated when blood glucose levels rise after a meal. It helps us realize when we have had enough to eat and are no longer hungry. Damage to this area causes a person to eat too much (again, especially carbohydrates) and eventually results in obesity.

The Hypothalamus and Circadian Rhythms

Many physiological functions fluctuate in a regular day-to-day cycle, called a circadian rhythm. These rhythms are controlled by neurons in the suprachiasmatic nucleus (SCN), which is sometimes referred to as the "master clock" of the body. Information about the light/dark cycle reaches the SCN through a direct projection from the retina. The SCN controls the release of other hypothalamic hormones that influence daily activities such as eating, drinking, and sleeping. Daily fluctuations in cortisol secretion are controlled by projections of the SCN to the paraventricular nucleus, which sends projections to sympathetic preganglionic neurons that synapse on the adrenal medulla. Secretion of melatonin is controlled by descending projections from the paraventricular nucleus to the sympathetic preganglionic neurons in the superior cervical ganglion, which projects to the pineal gland. The pineal gland, located on the surface of the midbrain just in front of the cerebellum, controls seasonal rhythms through its release of melatonin. In response to signals sent from the SCN through this indirect pathway, melatonin is secreted at night, with more being secreted on longer nights, such as during the winter.

THE HYPOTHALAMUS AND THE AUTONOMIC NERVOUS SYSTEM

In addition to its role in regulating the endocrine system, the hypothalamus also plays a key role in controlling the autonomic nervous system. There are three groups of neurons in the paraventricular nucleus. The group closest to the third ventricle produces corticotropin-releasing hormone, a second group produces oxytocin and vasopressin, and a third group sends projections through a descending pathway to the brainstem and spinal cord.

Although the third group of neurons does not project to the posterior pituitary lobe, these neurons release the peptide neurotransmitters oxytocin and vasopressin, along with glutamate. Their axons descend in the median forebrain bundle, which they leave in the brainstem to synapse on parasympathetic nuclei there or continue in a lateral pathway to synapse on the parasympathetic and sympathetic preganglionic neurons in the spinal cord. As you will recall, the sympathetic preganglionic neurons are located in the intermediolateral spinal cord in the thoracic and lumbar regions, and the parasympathetic neurons are located in cranial nerve nuclei in the brainstem and the sacral intermediolateral spinal cord. Neurons in the lateral hypothalamus, the posterior hypothalamus, and the dorsomedial hypothalamic nucleus also send projections through the descending pathway as well as to brainstem nuclei. Some hypothalamic areas project through the dorsal longitudinal fasciculus, which descends more medially near the ventricular system.

HYPOTHALAMUS AND STRESS RESPONSE

Stressors are stimuli that the brain perceives as a threat to physiological balance and normal functioning (homeostasis). Physical stressors include extreme temperatures, trauma, hypoglycemia, severe hypotension, and exercise. Psychological stressors include situations that produce negative emotions, such as fear and anxiety, or that require intense mental effort. Both types of stressors can trigger the **stress response**—a coordinated series of physiological reactions that gets the body ready to cope with the perceived threat. Short-term activation of the stress response helps preserve homeostasis. However, long-term activation of the stress response can be destructive.

During the stress response, the noradrenergic system, the sympathetic nervous system, and the **hypothalamic-pituito-adrenal (HPA) axis** become active. A projection from the central nucleus of the amygdala to the locus coeruleus is thought to activate the noradrenergic system, which has an activating effect on widespread areas of the brain and spinal cord, including the preganglionic sympathetic neurons.

The paraventricular hypothalamic nucleus, which plays an important role in the stress response, is activated by inputs from the amygdala, lateral hypothalamus, locus coeruleus, prefrontal cortex, and hippocampus. A group of neurons in the paraventricular nucleus of the hypothalamus is responsible for activating the sympathetic nervous system, which then releases norepinephrine that stimulates beta-adrenergic receptors in the cell membranes of the tissues and organs they innervate (including the heart and blood vessels). There are two exceptions to this general rule. Sympathetic postganglionic terminals connected to sweat glands release acetylcholine to bind with receptors on the postsynaptic membrane. The adrenal medulla (which is considered to be a sympathetic ganglion) is also activated by cholinergic nicotinic receptors rather than beta-adrenergic receptors. Secretory cells of the adrenal medulla then release norepinephrine and epinephrine into the bloodstream.

Activation of the sympathetic nervous system increases blood pressure and heart rate, dilates the pupils, shifts blood circulation to the brain and muscles, slows digestion, increases breathing rate, releases glucose from the liver and fatty acids from adipose (fatty) tissue, and decreases insulin production by the pancreas. Since all tissues except the brain need insulin to use glucose, the reduced amount of insulin lets the brain have a larger share of the circulating glucose available. All of these physiological changes get the body ready for "fight or flight," and prepare it to cope with threatening situations.

Another group of neurons in the paraventricular nucleus synthesizes corticotropin-releasing hormone (CRH). This hormone triggers the activation of the HPA axis by stimulating the production and release of ACTH by the anterior pituitary. ACTH, in turn, travels through the bloodstream to the adrenal cortex, where it stimulates the production and release of cortisol. Like norepinephrine and epinephrine, cortisol mobilizes the body's energy stores.

NEUROIMMUNE INTERACTIONS

The autonomic nervous system, which links the brain to the immune system, innervates the bone marrow, thymus gland, spleen, and lymph nodes. Both parasympathetic and sympathetic fibers connect to these immune organs. Neurotransmitter receptors for norepinephrine, epinephrine, dopamine, acetylcholine, serotonin, opioids, and GABA are found on leukocytes (white blood cells) and on lymphoid organs. Norepinephrine and epinephrine produced by the sympathetic nervous system during the stress response suppress the immune system. Acetylcholine, on the other hand, which is produced by the parasympathetic nervous system, stimulates the immune response.

Neurons in many brain regions have cytokine receptors. Cytokines, or immunotransmitters, are chemical messengers secreted by white blood cells in response to inflammation or invasion by foreign organisms. Cytokines enter the brain

WHAT IS AUTOIMMUNE DISEASE?

Autoimmune disease results when the body produces antibodies or immune cells that attack the body's own cells. These self-attacking antibodies and immune cells, also called autoantibodies and autoreactive T lymphocytes, respectively, cause damage to body tissues. A healthy immune system has the capacity to produce antibodies and T lymphocytes (also called T cells) that react to "self" instead of "foreign" proteins, a capacity that may be essential for normal functioning. However, with autoimmune disease, the inhibitory processes that prevent the immune system from producing too many of these autoreactive antibodies and cells are somehow disrupted. Development of autoimmune disease can be triggered by viral infections, certain drugs, hormones, environmental factors, and even sunlight, as in the case of systemic lupus erythematosus. The chemical element mercury, which is found in dental fillings and vaccine preparations, has also been implicated. More than 80 autoimmune diseases affect over 10 million Americans, 75% of whom are female. In most autoimmune diseases, a protein specific to a certain organ or tissue is targeted, but in some, such as systemic lupus erythematosus, the protein targeted is widespread enough that an inflammatory response takes place throughout the entire body. Autoimmune diseases of the nervous system include multiple sclerosis and myasthenia gravis. Scientists have found evidence that autoimmune processes may cause other dysfunctions of the nervous system, including obsessive-compulsive disorder, schizophrenia, and Alzheimer's disease. It is becoming apparent that having a healthy immune system is essential to having a healthy nervous system.

through membrane transporters. Neurons, microglia, and astrocytes also produce cytokines. Increased levels of cytokines resulting from infection or inflammation can affect the release of neurotransmitters in the brain. When cytokines are used to treat cancers, neurodegenerative diseases, and infections, they cause negative behavioral and neurological effects, such as memory problems, depression, paranoia, agitation, and impaired motor coordination.

CONNECTIONS

Through its control of pituitary gland secretion and the autonomic nervous system, the tiny hypothalamus has far-reaching effects on maintaining the homeostasis of body functions and on the body's reaction to stress. The hypothalamus and the secretion of the hormones it controls also regulate eating, drinking, and reproductive behavior. Circadian rhythms, or daily patterns of fluctuation in body rhythms, including the sleep/wake cycle, are under the control of the hypothalamus. Innervation of immune organs by the autonomic nervous system and the presence of receptors for neurotransmitters on immune cells and organs show the interaction between the immune system and the nervous system. Since nerve cells have receptors for cytokines, or immunotransmitters, it is apparent that this is a two-way interaction. Not only does the nervous system regulate the functions of the immune system, but the immune system, through its own set of chemical messengers, affects brain functions, including mood and cognition.

9

Sleep and Wakefulness

You may not think about it often, but sleep is a very important part of your life. Most people spend one-third of their entire lives sleeping! Many people think that the brain is inactive during sleep, but they're mistaken. In fact, sleep is an active, highly regulated process. Although we have less awareness of and responses to environmental stimuli while we sleep, most of the brain's activities do not change. Some studies suggest that the 90-minute cycles that occur during sleep may be part of an overall rest-activity cycle that occurs throughout the 24-hour day. This phenomenon was named the **basic rest-activity cycle** (**BRAC**) by American scientist Nathaniel Kleitman (1895–1999), who set up the first sleep research laboratory and is considered the "father of sleep research." Other studies have emphasized the role of a **circadian pacemaker** in the regulation of the sleep/wake cycle and its **entrainment**, or synchronization, with the light/dark pattern over a 24-hour period.

Although scientists have made great progress in understanding sleep over the last few decades, the reasons we sleep are not yet completely understood. At one time, experts believed that sleep's only purpose was to give the body physical rest and restoration. Studies of the biochemical changes that occur during sleep, however, suggest that this is not the case. Scientists found that a person's level of physical activity during the day does not correlate with the amount of deep sleep he or she gets that night. The amount of mental activity during the day, however, *does* relate to the amount of deep sleep we get at night. Currently, there is a growing consensus that the reason we sleep is to rest and restore the brain—not the body.

AROUSAL AND WAKEFULNESS

A fiber system called the **ascending reticular activating system,** or **ARAS,** helps control arousal and wakefulness (Figure 9.1). The ARAS ascends from nuclei in the brainstem. In addition to the brainstem neurons that contribute to the ARAS, there are wake-promoting areas in both the forebrain and the

NATHANIEL KLEITMAN: THE FATHER OF SLEEP RESEARCH

Nathaniel Kleitman, popularly known as the father of sleep research, set up the first sleep lab soon after he joined the faculty at the University of Chicago in 1925. His first major book on sleep, called *Sleep and Wakefulness*, was published in 1939. It is still an important work in sleep research.

Kleitman did use volunteers from the university for some of his experiments, but his main subjects were often members of his own family. From the time they were infants, Kleitman meticulously studied the sleeping habits of his two daughters. Once, Kleitman himself deliberately stayed awake for 180 hours to study the effects of sleep deprivation.

Kleitman is particularly noted for his important discoveries. Along with some of the students who helped him, Kleitman was the first to report the existence of REM (rapid eye movement) sleep, and was the first to measure eye movement and use electroencephalograms to chart the stages of sleep.

Kleitman, who was born in Russia in 1895 and became an American citizen in 1918, had a long career and an even longer life. He died in 1999 at the age of 104!

Source: "Nathaniel Kleitman, 1895–1999." The University of Chicago Hospitals. Available online at *http://www.uchospitals.edu/news/1999/ 19990816-kleitman.php.*

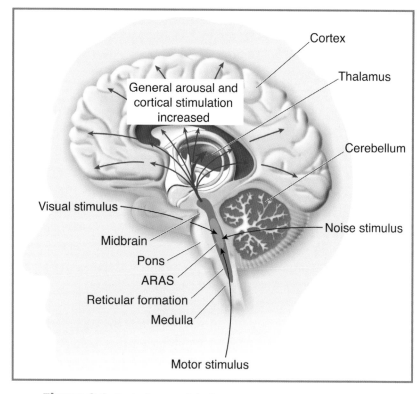

Figure 9.1 Brainstem nuclei whose axons make up the ascending reticular activating system (ARAS) include the locus coeruleus (norepinephrine), the raphe nuclei (serotonin), the ventral tegmental area (dopamine), and the pediculopontine tegmental (PPT) and laterodorsal tegmental (LDT) nuclei (acetylcholine). The ARAS causes activation, or arousal, of the cerebral cortex both by direct projections to the cortex and indirectly through relays in the thalamus, posterior hypothalamus, and septal nuclei.

hypothalamus. Also promoting wakefulness and arousal are cholinergic neurons in the basal nucleus of Meynert in the basal forebrain, as well as histaminergic neurons of the posterior hypothalamus. Hypocretin, or orexin, neurons located around the fornix in the lateral hypothalamus project widely in the brain and to the spinal cord. Orexins, which also influence eating behavior, seem to be important in keeping us alert. A deficiency in orexin transmission, possibly due to an autoimmune reaction that deactivates or destroys orexin receptors, has been suggested as one of the causes of **narcolepsy**, a disorder in which a person is constantly sleepy during the daytime.

Cholinergic neurons in the basal forebrain connect directly to the cerebral cortex and activate it. Fibers from the brainstem **pedunculopontine tegmental nuclei** (**PPT**) and **laterodorsal tegmental nuclei** (**LDT**) project through the ARAS. They relay first in the thalamus, sending fibers to most of the thalamic nuclei. These fibers release acetylcholine, which stimulates the intralaminar thalamic nuclei directly and also releases them from inhibition by inhibiting the GABAergic (activated by GABA) neurons of the reticular thalamic nuclei. PPT/LDT neurons are active during both wakefulness and REM sleep, which we will discuss later in this chapter.

When we are awake, cholinergic and other ARAS inputs to the thalamic relay nuclei enhance thalamic transmission, which keeps the cerebral cortex continuously active. As you will recall, fibers that take in sensory information from all senses except smell relay their messages first in the thalamus before sending them on to the cerebral cortex. Collaterals, or branches, of these fibers also end in the reticular formation. When the ARAS is inhibited, transmission of sensory information through the thalamus is inhibited. This produces the reduction in awareness that is typical of sleep.

SLEEP

An opposing influence from the anterior hypothalamus promotes sleep. When the anterior hypothalamus is electrically stimulated, it induces sleep. The pupils of the eye constrict and there is a decrease in heart rate, blood pressure, and body temperature. A group of GABAergic neurons in the ventrolateral preoptic nucleus (VLPO), which is located just to the side of the optic chiasm, projects to the serotonergic and noradrenergic nuclei in the brainstem. These GABAergic neurons promote sleep by inhibiting the activity of these nuclei. Galanin, which is released along with GABA from these neurons, also promotes sleep. Little direct input from the SCN reaches the VLPO, but indirect input comes from a number of areas that are innervated by the SCN. GABAergic fibers from the VPLO nucleus also terminate on histaminergic neurons in the posterior hypothalamus. Like the locus coeruleus (adrenergic) and the raphe nuclei (serotonergic), the histaminergic nuclei are most active during wakefulness, less active during NREM (non-rapid eye movement) sleep, and inactive during REM (rapid eye movement) sleep. Neurons in the preoptic nucleus, some of which secrete serotonin and adenosine, also promote sleep.

Sleepiness appears to be regulated by homeostatic and circadian mechanisms. How long and how deeply we sleep after we have experienced a sleep loss is proportional to the length of time we were awake. That is, sleep varies with the duration of prior wakefulness.

There are two basic types of sleep: **synchronized**, or **nonREM sleep**, and **desynchronized**, or **REM sleep**, which is named after the characteristic eye movements that occur during this type of sleep. About every 90 minutes, the sleep cycle shifts from nonREM sleep to REM sleep. Ranging from 5 to 30 minutes, periods of REM sleep get longer each time the body reaches the REM stage during the night (Figure 9.2).

Scientists monitor brain activity during sleep by attaching electrodes to a person's scalp. The brain waves that appear are recorded as an **electroencephalogram (EEG)**. Electrodes attached near the eyes monitor eye movements and record the results as an **electro-oculogram (EOG)**. Muscle activity is monitored with electrodes attached to the chin and recorded as an **electromyogram (EMG)**.

When we are awake, there are two main types of electrical activity in our brains: alpha rhythms and beta rhythms. **Alpha activity** occurs when we are resting quietly (usually with our

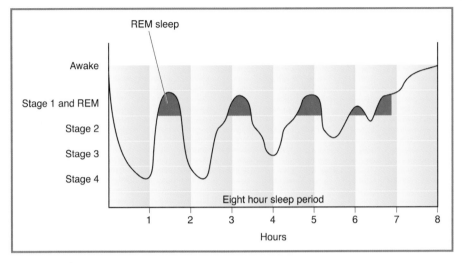

Figure 9.2 On average, the sleep cycle repeats every 90 minutes, resulting in 4 or 5 cycles during the night. As the night progresses, the time spent in Stages 3 and 4 decreases. In fact, most deep sleep occurs during the first half of the night. During the rest of the night, Stage 2 sleep and REM sleep increase more during each sleep cycle. Meaningful stimuli (like someone saying your name) will awaken you during REM sleep, but only loud noises will awaken you from Stage 4 sleep. You will be groggy and confused if awakened from deep sleep but alert and attentive if awakened during REM sleep.

eyes closed). During alpha activity, regular waves occur at a frequency of 8 to 12 cycles per second. **Beta activity**, on the other hand, occurs when we are alert, attentive, or actively thinking. Waves during this type of activity are irregular and of low amplitude and occur at a frequency of 13 to 30 cycles per second. The more active the brain is, the lower is the amplitude and the higher is the frequency (speed) of the brain waves that are shown by the EEG.

STAGES OF SLEEP

There are four stages of NREM sleep. As drowsiness sets in, we enter Stage 1, which is a transition from wakefulness to sleep. This sleep stage is characterized by alpha activity and some theta activity, which has a frequency of 3.5–7.5 cycles per second. In Stage 1, we drift in and out of sleep—although the actual changeover from wakefulness to sleep happens instantaneously, not gradually. During this stage, our muscles start to relax and our breathing gets slower. We are still conscious enough, however, to become quickly alert if we hear a noise or are disturbed in some other way.

During Stage 2 of NREM sleep, an EEG will show our brain activity as irregular. This stage of sleep is characterized by sleep spindles and K complexes as well as some theta activity. Sleep spindles are bursts of activity at a frequency of 12 to 14 cycles per second that last less than a second and occur about 2 to 5 times a minute during all 4 stages of NREM sleep. K complexes also take place during this stage, and *only* during this stage. K complexes are sudden, high-amplitude waves that occur about once every minute, and also in response to noises. While in Stage 2, a person's eyes move slowly from side to side. Although the sleeper can still be roused fairly easily, it would take a much louder noise to wake a person from Stage 2 sleep than from Stage 1.

Stages 3 and 4 are known as **slow-wave sleep**, or **deep sleep**. They are characterized by the presence of **delta activity**—high-amplitude waves with a frequency of less than 3.5 cycles per minute. Delta activity makes up between 20 and 50% of the Stage 3 EEG and over 50% of the Stage 4 EEG. A person in Stage 3 sleep is transitioning into deep sleep and becoming more and more difficult to arouse. People who are awakened during deep sleep usually do not report dreaming, but if they do, the dreams are usually nightmares.

Our blood pressure, heart rate, systemic vascular resistance, and cardiac output remain regular but decline as we move to later stages of NREM sleep. Parasympathetic activity increases, while sympathetic activity decreases. Because the heart does not have to work as hard, it can replenish its cardiac metabolic stores. This replenishment is necessary to keep the heart muscle healthy.

While we sleep, we no longer have voluntary control over our breathing. Thermoregulatory responses (activities that regulate body temperature), such as sweating and shivering, remain active.

REM SLEEP

About 90 minutes after the onset of Stage 1 sleep, the EEG changes suddenly to resemble the irregular pattern of the waking EEG. REM sleep is called "paradoxical sleep" because the electrical activity of the brain is similar to that seen when we are awake than what we show at other stages of sleep. People awakened from REM sleep report vivid, story-like dreams. During REM sleep, we lose our muscle tone—which protects us from acting out our dreams and possibly hurting ourselves.

During slow-wave (deep) sleep, peripheral blood flow is reduced except to the heart and skeletal muscles. Heart rate varies a lot; it may have very slow or very fast episodes. Breathing is irregular and activity of the diaphragm increases. The metabolic rate either increases or shows no change. Cerebral blood flow and general metabolism are both similar to the levels at which they commonly are when we are awake.

Scientists continue to debate whether sleep plays a role in memory consolidation, and if so, which stages of sleep are most important. There is some evidence that slow-wave (deep) sleep and, to a lesser extent, REM sleep, may be involved in the consolidation of certain types of memory, particularly procedural memory.

CIRCADIAN INFLUENCES ON SLEEP

Whether we sleep or wake depends on the interplay of several neurotransmitter systems of the brain as well as the influences of hypothalamic nuclei (Figure 9.3). Sleep/wake cycle timing

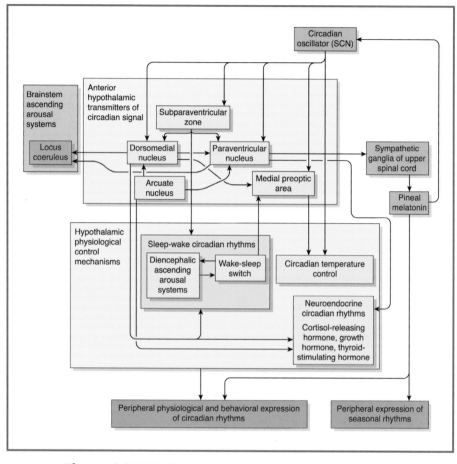

Figure 9.3 This flow chart depicts the interactions of the suprachiasmatic nucleus (SCN) directly and indirectly with other hypothalamic nuclei and indirectly with the pineal gland in the circadian control of the sleep/wake cycle and physiological functions. Feedback from the pineal gland, which produces melatonin, is also shown. This feedback is thought to have a modulatory influence on the SCN's control of circadian rhythms.

is regulated by the suprachiasmatic nucleus. Firing rates of suprachiasmatic neurons are low at night and high during the day. There are projections from the SCN to the thalamus, the basal forebrain, and the subventricular zone and dorsomedial nucleus of the hypothalamus. Direct projections to the hypocretin/orexin neurons may be involved in the SCN's promotion of wakefulness.

Melatonin secretion, which is low during the light phase and high during the dark phase, is also regulated by the SCN. Projections from the SCN terminate in the hypothalamic subventricular zone, from which neurons project through the median forebrain bundle to synapse on preganglionic autonomic neurons in the spinal cord. Postganglionic fibers from the superior cervical ganglion then project to the pineal gland, from which melatonin is secreted. Although the pineal gland appears to be the primary source of circulating melatonin, melatonin is also synthesized in the gastrointestinal tract and the retina, as well as a number of other places. It circulates in the cerebrospinal fluid and in the blood and reaches all areas of the brain and body. Under the control of the SCN, it acts as an indirect circadian messenger and helps to synchronize sleep with the day/night cycle. Once secreted, melatonin has an inhibitory effect on the SCN and its promotion of wakefulness.

Plasma concentrations of melatonin start to rise between 9 and 10 P.M., peak between 2 and 4 A.M., and then decline until the low daytime levels are reached between 7 and 9 A.M. Exposure to light can cause a phase change in melatonin secretion. Prolonged exposure to light during the evening hours delays the secretion of melatonin, and prolonged exposure to darkness during the morning hours extends melatonin secretion. Brief light exposures during the night will temporarily decrease melatonin secretion. Melatonin levels range from very low in infants to maximum levels in children around age 3. This is followed by a decline, which is pronounced during puberty. The decline in melatonin levels is complete by age 20 to 30, after which they remain stable. There is a 20-fold variation between individuals in the amount of melatonin that they secrete.

Taking vitamin B$_6$ or tryptophan causes the brain to produce more melatonin. When people who have insomnia (an inability to fall or remain asleep) take melatonin, they often get some relief.

DISORDERS OF SLEEP

Insomnia, the most common sleep complaint, is actually a symptom rather than a disorder. Although most people experience insomnia at some point in their lives, it can also be a component of such conditions as Alzheimer's disease or African sleeping sickness. According to surveys, 10 to 15% of adults in the developed world have insomnia at any given time, and each year, one-third of the population experiences insomnia to some degree.

Excessive daytime sleepiness is also a symptom as opposed to a condition in and of itself. It occurs in about 5% of adults.

SLEEPWALKING

Somnambulism, or sleepwalking, is a state of incomplete arousal during Stage 3 or 4 of slow wave sleep. It is most common in young adults and children and may even be seen in infancy—the child will crawl around while sleeping. Onset of sleepwalking usually occurs after 18 months. It is most prevalent between ages 11 and 12; some 16.7% of people this age sleepwalk. More males than females are sleepwalkers. Sleepwalking that begins before age 9 may continue into adulthood. Episodes may range in frequency from less than once a month to almost every night in severe cases. Fever, noise in the sleep environment, stress, a distended bladder, and pain can bring on an episode. Most cases of sleepwalking do not result in physical harm, but there have been cases of physical injury and a few cases of violent behavior. Safety precautions for vulnerable individuals include getting adequate rest, relaxing before going to bed, using a ground floor bedroom, placing furniture in front of large windows, and ensuring that doors and windows are not easy to open.

It is most common in shift workers (people who work at night or at other unusual hours), young adults, and the elderly, and is associated with snoring, sleep deprivation, and the use of hypnotic (sleep-inducing) drugs.

There are several types of sleepiness. Subalertness is a reduced arousal state that varies with the circadian rhythm phase and the quality and duration of the last period of sleep. Drowsiness is sleepiness during the day that does not necessarily result in sleep. Micro sleeps are sleep episodes that occur during the day and last only a few seconds.

Narcolepsy is a disorder in which REM sleep occurs during waking hours. There is some evidence that it happens because of a lack of orexin/hypocretin, possibly due to a genetic mutation or an autoimmune reaction. Brain damage can also cause narcolepsy. The sleep attack is its primary symptom. A sleep attack is an overwhelming need to sleep that usually happens when conditions are monotonous. It results in 2 to 5 minutes of REM sleep and leaves the person feeling refreshed. In cataplexy (another symptom of narcolepsy), sleep atonia—or sleep paralysis, a component of REM sleep—occurs suddenly. The person falls to the ground and lies there for up to several minutes without losing awareness. Cataplexy usually results from a sudden physical movement in response to an unexpected event or to strong emotions such as anger or laughter. **Hypnagogic hallucinations** occur when REM dreaming accompanies sleep paralysis while the person is awake just before or after sleep.

REM sleep behavior disorder is a condition in which normal sleep paralysis does not occur and the person acts out the vivid dreams he or she has during REM sleep. It is most common during the first round of REM sleep of the night. Like narcolepsy, it appears to have a genetic component and can also result from brain damage. The movements the sufferer makes can range from twitches to arm flailing, talking, running, jumping, or more aggressive actions. It is most common after age 50 and is four times more common in males than in females.

CONNECTIONS

Sleep is an active process, as scientists have demonstrated by observing electrical activity on an EEG during the various stages of sleep. In the 90-minute sleep cycle, four progressively deepening stages of NREM sleep come before an episode of REM sleep. Also known as paradoxical sleep because the brain's electrical activity is so similar to that of the waking state, REM sleep is characterized by vivid dreams and a loss of muscle tone. Wakefulness is promoted by serotonergic and noradrenergic nuclei in the brainstem and by histaminergic neurons in the posterior hypothalamus. GABAergic neurons in the VLPO nucleus in the anterior hypothalamus promote sleep by inhibiting these neurons. Cholinergic neurons in the basal forebrain promote wakefulness, and the PPT/LDT nuclei in the brainstem promote REM sleep. This latter set of cholinergic neurons are inhibited by serotinergic and noradrenergic projections, which become silent during REM sleep. Orexin neurons in the hypothalamus promote wakefulness by projecting to cholinergic, histaminergic, and monoaminergic neurons.

Timing of the sleep/wake cycle is regulated by the suprachiasmatic nucleus of the thalamus. Melatonin helps synchronize the sleep/wake cycle with the day/night cycle. Sleep deprivation results in suppression of immune functions. Infections promote sleep as do increased levels of cytokines in the absence of infection.

The production of growth hormone, prolactin, TSH, and cortisol are all regulated by the sleep/wake cycle. While the secretion of growth hormone and prolactin are primarily controlled by the sleep/wake cycle, cortisol secretion is somewhat influenced by sleep but is primarily under circadian control, and thyrotropin secretion has a circadian rhythm but is inhibited by sleep.

10

Diseases and Injuries of the Nervous System

Few of us will go through life without being affected, either personally or through a friend or relative, by some kind of disease or injury of the nervous system. What effect a nervous system disease or injury has depends greatly on the point in the neural pathway where it occurs. Some effects of injuries and disorders are so subtle that they are almost unnoticeable. Others can be devastating to a person's daily life.

DISEASE AND INJURY OF THE NEUROMUSCULAR SYSTEM

Diseases and disorders that affect the neuromuscular system can impair movement. Such conditions can be caused by viruses, environmental toxins, autoimmune responses, and side effects of medications. Some conditions are genetic, meaning that they result from a specific gene mutation or from a genetic predisposition (an increased susceptibility that runs in one's family). The effects of these diseases can be crippling and even lethal.

Neuromuscular Autoimmune Disease

Autoimmune diseases occur when the immune system attacks the body's own proteins as if they were foreign proteins. Myasthenia gravis is an autoimmune disorder in which antibodies to the nicotinic receptors at the neuromuscular junction are formed. These antibodies block the receptors and cause muscle weakness. Symptoms include drooping eyelids, double vision, problems swallowing and talking, and general weakness and fatigue. This disorder affects 3 to 4 people out of 100,000 and is usually progressive, ultimately ending in death.

Multiple sclerosis (MS) is an autoimmune disease in which antibodies break down the myelin layer that surrounds the axons of the brain and spinal cord. This destruction of the myelin makes the nerve impulses move more slowly through the nerve fibers. Symptoms of MS can include visual problems, fatigue, pain, numbness, tingling, difficulty walking, depression, bowel or bladder problems, sexual dysfunction, and problems with attention, memory, and problem-solving. Less common symptoms include tremor, speech problems, impaired hearing, difficulty swallowing, and a lack of coordination. Several viruses (including those that cause German measles, mononucleosis, and canine distemper) have been implicated as possible causes of multiple sclerosis, either because they destroy the myelin layer or trigger an autoimmune response. The connection of these viruses to multiple sclerosis has not yet been proven, however. Genetic factors that make a person more vulnerable to certain environmental factors may also play a role. Multiple sclerosis can be mild, moderate, or severe—the course and symptoms vary a great deal from person to person. Despite the potential seriousness of the disease, most people with multiple sclerosis now live out 95% of their normal lifespan.

Basal Ganglia Disorders

Parkinson's disease is a movement disorder caused by the degeneration of neurons in the substantia nigra that produce dopamine (Figure 10.1). Usually, Parkinson's disease appears in people between the ages of 50 and 60. Analysis of brain tissue from Parkinson's patients who have died has shown a

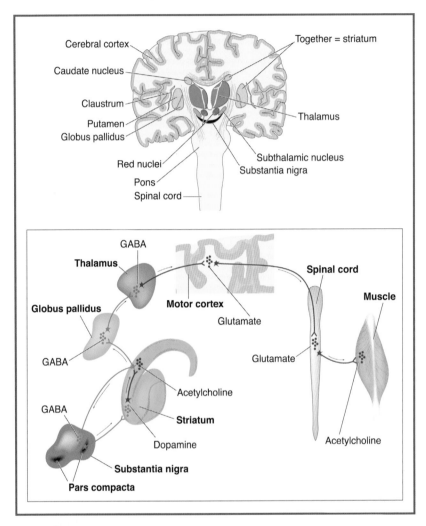

Figure 10.1 Except for the claustrum, whose function is unknown, the structures (or portions thereof) shown in the upper figure play a part in the control of movement. The lower figure shows how the basal ganglia interact to help control movement indirectly through their effect on the thalamus. In Parkinson's disease, up to 80% of the dopaminergic neurons in the substantia nigra are destroyed. Cholinergic interneurons in the striatum, which are normally inhibited by dopamine, become overactive. Cholinergic overactivity in the striatum is considered the primary cause of the rigidity and tremors of Parkinson's disease.

loss of the black pigment that is normally seen in the substantia nigra. This pigment is called neuromelanin and is a by-product of dopamine metabolism. Symptoms of Parkinson's disease include problems with initiating movements, slowness in movement, rigidity due to increased muscle tone, and tremors of the hands, arms, and head when they are at rest. Problems with posture, equilibrium, and the function of the autonomic nervous system may also be present. The sufferer speaks slowly and in a monotone, handwriting becomes very small, and facial expressions are lost.

Degeneration of neurons (particularly those that produce acetylcholine and GABA) of the putamen and caudate nucleus results in a disorder called Huntington's chorea. Wasting (atrophy) of the tissues of the cerebral cortex also occurs. Symptoms, which include involuntary movements (particularly of the limbs), usually appear when the victim is between age 35 and 45, but can occur in the early twenties and sometimes even during childhood. Progressive dementia and emotional problems, including depression, can be part of this disorder. The disease, which has been traced to a mutation of a gene located on chromosome 4, is hereditary, and it always ends in death. Children of parents who have Huntington's chorea have a 50% chance of inheriting this gene.

Prolonged use of antipsychotic drugs can cause a largely irreversible movement disorder in 50% or more of patients. Symptoms of this disorder include facial tics, grimacing, rapid eye blinking, peculiar gestures, cheek puffing, tongue protrusion, and lip pursing. Writhing movements of the trunk and hands are sometimes present as well. Because the basal ganglia, which are impaired in this disorder, play a role in higher cognitive functions, many tardive dyskinesia patients also develop **dementia**. Scientists theorize that the disorder results when dopaminergic receptors in the postsynaptic membrane overcompensate for the inhibition of dopaminergic receptors by antipsychotic drugs.

Cerebellar Disorders

Damage to the cerebellum results in loss of coordination and reduced muscle tone. The specific symptoms depend on which area of the cerebellum is harmed. One common symptom is **ataxia**, or "drunken gait." Goose-stepping, or high stepping, may occur. **Movement decomposition**, in which smooth motions decompose into a jerky series of discrete movements, may be present. Other symptoms of cerebellar damage are **dysmetria**, or overshooting of targets (for example, when the person points), and **intention tremor**, or tremor while a limb or extremity is in motion. **Dysdiadochokinesia**, the inability to produce rapid alternating movements (such as finger tapping or quick turns while walking), may occur. If the cerebellum is damaged on just one side, only that side of the body is affected.

Motor Neuron Disease

Amyotrophic lateral sclerosis (ALS), also known as Lou Gehrig's disease, results when the motor neurons in the brain, brainstem, and spinal cord degenerate and the lateral corticospinal tracts deteriorate. Symptoms include hyperactive reflexes, atrophy of muscles, muscle weakness, and **fasciculations**, or spasms of the fibers of a single motor unit. People who get this disease usually live for only 3 to 5 years.

Apraxias are problems performing learned skilled movements that result from damage to the frontal or parietal lobes or the corpus callosum. Limb apraxia involves difficulty performing tasks with the fingers, hands, or arms. Speech impairments due to problems moving the muscles needed to speak are called apraxic agraphia. Problems with drawing and building or assembling objects may result from constructional apraxia, which is caused by damage to the right cerebral hemisphere, particularly the right parietal lobe.

Epilepsy

Epilepsy is a neurological condition in which recurring seizures are the main symptom. It affects about 0.4 to 0.8% of the population. A seizure occurs when a large group of neurons fires together repetitively in synchrony. Everyone's brain is able to produce a seizure under certain conditions. Some people may have lower thresholds for seizure activity and may therefore be more susceptible to having spontaneous seizures. Seizures can be triggered in vulnerable individuals by emotional stress, sleep deprivation, alcohol withdrawal, menstrual cycle phases, and sometimes, specific stimuli, such as strobe lights. Seizures may also be caused by chemical stimuli, such as reduced levels of certain neurotransmitters (Figure 10.2). Seizure thresholds may be lowered in areas of the brain that have suffered damage from trauma, stroke, brain infection (such as meningitis or encephalitis), tumor, or neurodegenerative diseases.

Generalized epilepsy is a type of epilepsy in which large areas of both cerebral hemispheres seem to discharge at the same time. Most cases of generalized epilepsy begin before age 20. Focal epilepsy, which may begin at any age, is a type of epilepsy in which the electrical discharge that causes the seizure begins in one particular area in the brain—usually a place where an injury (from trauma, stroke, tumor, prenatal toxin exposure, or other cause) has previously occurred. The abnormal electrical discharge can remain fixed at its point of origin, or **locus**, or it can spread to the rest of the brain to become a generalized seizure.

SPINAL CORD INJURY

Approximately 11,000 cases of spinal cord injury (SCI) occur in the United States each year. There are a total of about 243,000 Americans living with spinal cord injuries today. The yearly figure does not include SCI incurred in fatal accidents. A little over half (53%) of SCIs occur in young adults, with

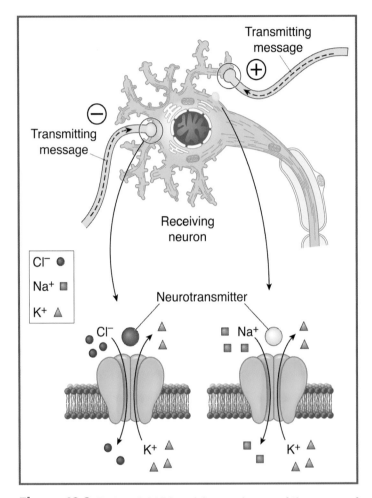

Figure 10.2 Reduced **GABA** activity may be one of the causes of some cases of epilepsy. Activation of the **GABA** receptor results in an influx of chlorine ions (Cl⁻) into the cell. This results in a hyper-polarization of the cell and a decrease in the probability of an action potential. (The influx of sodium ions (Na⁺) into a cell has the oppo-site effect of depolarization.) Under normal conditions, inhibitory GABAergic neurons keep excitatory glutamatergic neurons in check so that the brain is not overstimulated. In some epileptic brains, there may be reduced GABAergic transmission that may be due to lower levels of **GABA**, excessive deactivation of **GABA** by enzymes, or changes in binding properties of **GABA** receptors. However, this is just one of the possible causes of epilepsy.

32.6 years being the average age at the time of injury. Most SCIs (81.2%) occur in males. The primary causes of SCI are automobile accidents (40.9%), falls (22.4%), violence (21.6%), and sports (7.5%). SCI can also result from diseases of the spinal cord or vertebral column.

If the spinal column is fractured or displaced, it pinches the spinal cord and may cause contusion (bruising), along with edema (swelling) and hemorrhage (bleeding). SCI may affect neurons within the spinal cord as well as the ascending and descending fiber pathways that travel through it. The **level of injury** is the most caudal (bottommost) vertebral segment at which there is a decrease or absence of sensation and movement on both sides of the body. **Tetraplegia** (also known as **quadriplegia**) is a term used to describe an injury in the neck region. With tetraplegia, a person loses sensation and movement in all four limbs. **Paraplegia** is the term used to describe injuries in the rest of the spinal cord. Depending on the level of injury, movement and sensation may be impaired anywhere from the middle of the chest downward through the lower extremities. Approximately 51.7% of spinal cord injuries result in tetraplegia, and about 46.7% result in paraplegia.

Extensive damage to the spinal cord can result in a complete spinal cord injury, in which all sensation and movement is lost below the level of the injury. Complete injuries make up nearly half of all SCIs. How much movement and sensation is preserved in an incomplete SCI depends on where the injury is and which nerve pathways run through the damaged area. Most SCI patients experience a loss of bladder and bowel control and sexual dysfunction. Chronic pain may be a problem, even in the areas of the body where other sensation is lost. The person may also lose the ability to sweat, which leads to problems with temperature control.

There is usually little recovery of function after a complete SCI. With an incomplete SCI, any improvement that takes place usually begins within the first few days to the first 6 months after the injury. Most recovery of function occurs within the first year after the injury. If function is still absent after 1 to 2 years, the loss is usually permanent. There are exceptions to this general rule, however, including actor Christopher Reeve, whose efforts to find effective treatments for himself and others have stimulated research efforts in the field that hold promise for improved outcomes for SCI victims.

STROKE

About 700,000 incidents of stroke occur each year in the United States, causing over 200,000 deaths. This makes stroke the third leading cause of death after heart disease and cancer.

THE INSPIRING STORY OF CHRISTOPHER REEVE

Perhaps best known for portraying the comic book hero in the *Superman* movies, Christopher Reeve became famous and respected worldwide for a very different reason. After Reeve suffered a severe spinal cord injury during a horseback riding competition in 1995 that left him completely paralyzed from the neck down, he quickly became an international spokesman for research into ways to treat and perhaps someday cure spinal cord injuries. In 1999, Reeve founded the Christopher Reeve Paralysis Foundation (CRPS), which works to promote research and provides funding to improve the lives of people who have been disabled by SCI. As the CRPS Website explains, ". . . Reeve has not only put a human face on spinal cord injury but he has motivated neuroscientists around the world to conquer the most complex diseases of the brain and central nervous system." Sadly, Reeve died in October 2004 from complications of a pressure wound infection.

Source: "Christopher Reeve: Biography." Christopher Reeve Paralysis Foundation. Available online at *http://www.christopherreeve.org*.

Risk factors for stroke include age, high blood pressure, cardiac disease, diabetes mellitus, smoking, high cholesterol, excessive use of alcohol, atherosclerosis of arteries in the neck and limbs, previous transient "mini-strokes," oral contraceptive use, obesity, and lack of exercise.

The two basic types of stroke are **ischemic** (88% of all strokes) and **hemorrhagic** (12% of strokes). Ischemia is the interruption of the blood supply to a certain brain area, which deprives it of oxygen and glucose. Embolytic stroke is the most common form of ischemic stroke. An **embolism** occurs when a blood clot formed somewhere else in the body blocks a blood vessel in the brain. Most such clots form during heart attacks, atrial fibrillation, or as a result of a dysfunction of the heart valves. Hemorrhagic stroke, on the other hand, causes blood to be released onto the surface of the brain (subdural hematoma), into the subarachnoid space, or into brain tissue. Subarachnoid hemorrhage occurs when one of the large arteries at the base of the brain ruptures and fills the subarachnoid space. This produces an increase in intracranial pressure that can result in unconsciousness or death. Intracerebral hemorrhage, most commonly caused by hypertension, results from the rupture of small arteries within the brain. This allows blood to leak into the brain tissue. Trauma and aneurysm (a condition caused by the ballooning and rupture of a weakened area in the wall of a blood vessel) are the most common causes of subarachnoid hemorrhage.

Symptoms of stroke depend on where and how severe the lesion is. A lesion in the front left cerebral hemisphere causes symptoms that can include weakness and loss of sensation in the right limb, aphasia, problems with the right visual field, and difficulties with writing, reading, and making calculations. If the lesion is in the front right hemisphere, similar symptoms can occur on the left side of the body. Rather than problems with reading and writing, however, the person will have trouble copying and drawing. Symptoms of a pure motor stroke, which results from a lesion in the internal capsule or the base of the pons, are unilateral weakness of the arm, leg, and face with no changes in visual, sensory, or cognitive functions. Pure sensory stroke due to a lesion to the thalamus (the relay station for the senses) results in unilateral numbness of the arm, leg, and face, with no weakness or visual or cognitive dysfunction. Different sets of symptoms may be present for lesions in other areas of the brain.

TRAUMATIC BRAIN INJURY

Traumatic brain injury (TBI) is damage to the brain that comes from some type of blow to the head or as a result of acceleration-deceleration forces. Each year, over 700,000 incidents of TBI occur in the United States, causing about 75,000 deaths and about 90,000 long-term disabilities, including 20,000 cases of epilepsy. TBI is responsible for one-third to one-half of all traumatic deaths and is the major cause of disabling symptoms in people under the age of 45. It is also the leading cause of death for children and adolescents. Approximately half of TBI cases result from motor vehicle accidents or other transportation-related injuries. Other leading causes of TBI include falls, firearms, and work-related injuries (particularly military). Sports-related injuries are another major cause of TBI. The use of seat belts, helmets, and child restraints has reduced the incidence of TBI—except for those resulting from firearms, which are on the increase.

Diffuse axonal injury (DAI) is the major cause of injury in up to 50% of TBIs that require hospitalization, and it also causes 35% of TBI-related deaths. If the victim loses consciousness, doctors assume that DAI has occurred. There does not have to be physical impact for DAI to result. Whiplash from an automobile accident, for example, can be severe enough to kill a person. Rapid acceleration and deceleration of the brain causes a shearing motion of the axonal cytoplasm. This can damage the axons and cause them to degenerate, a process which may continue for months to years after the injury. Neuronal cell bodies and glial cells may also degenerate due to secondary processes.

DEMENTIAS

Dementia is a disease primarily associated with aging. It is rarely seen in people younger than 60. The various types of dementia are characterized by the pathological changes in brain tissue that occur and by the resulting cognitive and behavioral changes. Since dementias represent a progressive deterioration of the brain, they are all eventually fatal. As the number of people over the age of 60 increases (due to improvements in health care and lifestyles), the number of people with some form of dementia will grow, making these disorders a major challenge to medical professionals and an important focus for research efforts.

Alzheimer's disease (AD) is perhaps the best known and most feared type of dementia. It currently affects 4 million people in the United States alone, and is the most common form of dementia in people over age 60. A small percentage of Alzheimer cases are seen in patients under 60 (these cases are known as early onset Alzheimer's disease) and are thought to result from specific inherited mutations in genes located on chromosomes 1, 14, and 21. Patients with Down's syndrome develop Alzheimer's disease by the time they reach middle age. Late onset Alzheimer's disease, which represents the rest of Alzheimer's disease cases, attacks victims older than 60. It is believed to result from susceptibility to one or more risk factors, including environmental factors. The length of time between diagnosis and death can vary from 5 to 20 years.

The progressive dementia of Alzheimer's disease begins as a subtle change in declarative memory, caused by gradual damage to the brain structures involved in cognitive processes. As the disease progresses, symptoms become more pronounced. Mood swings, language deterioration, personality changes, poor judgment, and confusion become more severe as the disease progresses. Eventually, the patient loses the ability to speak, becomes bedridden, and dies. MRI studies have revealed that neurodegeneration in Alzheimer's disease begins in the entorhinal cortex and spreads to the hippocampus and other limbic areas of the temporal lobe, then moves on to higher-order association cortices (Figure 10.3). Sensorimotor and sensory areas of the cortex are spared. The neuropathology of Alzheimer's is characterized by amyloid plaques and neuro-fibrillary tangles. Beta-amyloid protein is overproduced in Alzheimer's and is deposited between the neurons. Micro-tubules, which normally transport neurotransmitter down the axon, break apart, and their subunits accumulate as neurofibrillary tangles inside diseased neurons. Subunits of microfilaments, which normally provide structural sup-port to the cell, accumulate to form small structures called inclusion bodies.

Vascular dementia is the second most common type of dementia. It is caused by damage to the brain resulting from one large stroke or multiple small ones. Symptoms vary depending on where the lesion is located in the brain. Autop-sies of many patients who had vascular dementia also show the neuropathological changes that are associated with Alzheimer's disease. About 30% of Alzheimer's disease patients also have lesions caused by stroke.

Pick's Disease (PcD) is characterized by Pick bodies, cytoplasmic inclusions made up of tau protein fibrils, that range in size from one half to two times that of the nucleus and displace the nucleus in the opposite direction. It is also char-acterized by ballooned, or swollen, neurons, termed Pick cells. There is atrophy (or shrinking) of the frontal and/or temporal lobes, with or without atrophy of the parietal cortex. Behavioral and personality changes, such as aggressive-ness, agitation, disinhibition, apathy, impulsivity, and impaired judgment are early symptoms of PcD. **Anomia**, or difficulty finding words, is a language impairment that is

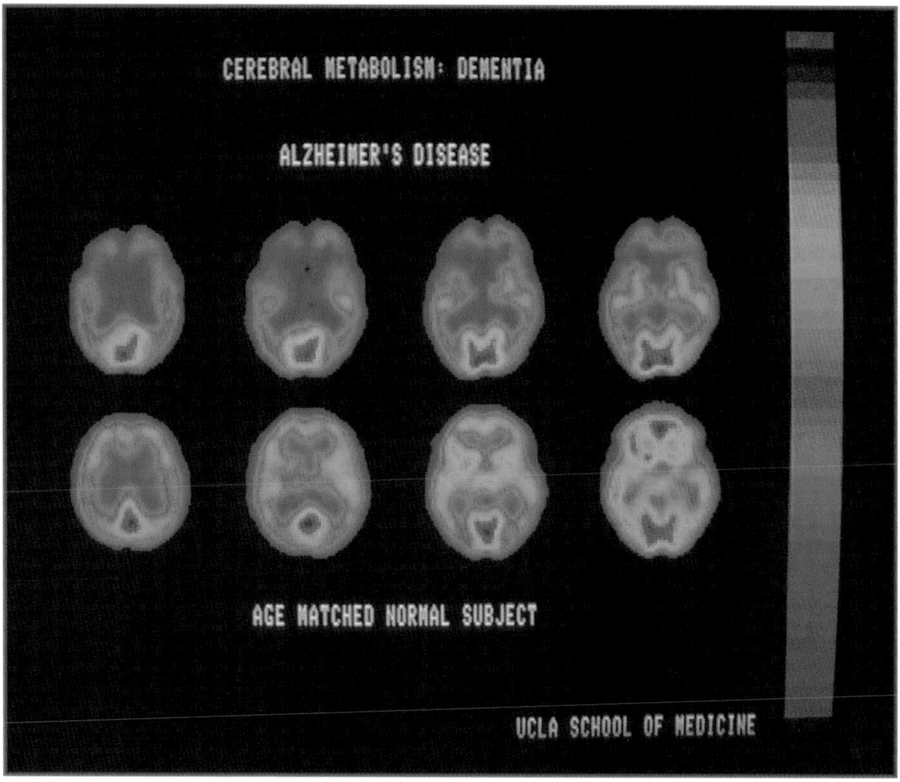

CEREBRAL METABOLISM: DEMENTIA

ALZHEIMER'S DISEASE

AGE MATCHED NORMAL SUBJECT

UCLA SCHOOL OF MEDICINE

Figure 10.3 Alzheimer's disease causes impairment of cognition (thinking). This concept is demonstrated by these PET scans taken during a research study of the brain of an Alzheimer's patient and healthy patient of the same age. Age-matched normal controls have higher levels of cerebral metabolism. The more active areas are "lit up" with color that changes with the intensity of the radioactivity, such as red for the most active areas, yellow for the next most active areas, and so on. A reduced level of cerebral metabolism is evidence of reduced activity of neurons. This lowered level of metabolism could be due to the loss of neurons that is characteristic of Alzheimer's. It could also be partly due to impaired function of remaining neurons.

present early in the disease. Explicit memory impairment, which is the primary initial symptom of Alzheimer's, with which PcD is sometimes confused in diagnosis, is less pronounced in Pick's disease, as is impairment of visuospatial function. As the disease progresses, all cognitive functions decline. A rapid decline in expressive language, resulting in aphasia, is diagnostic of PcD.

Prion diseases are neurodegenerative diseases caused by abnormally folded proteins called **prions**, also known as "slow viruses." Prions are resistant to enzymatic deactivation because they do not possess nucleic acids as do viruses and other infectious agents. When examined with a microscope, the brain of a person with prion disease is seen to have a spongiform encephalopathy, in which vacuoles (tiny, fluid-filled cavities) fill the neuronal cytoplasm and make the damaged tissue look porous like a sponge when viewed under the microscope. Symptoms may not appear for 1 to 20 years, but once the disease is active, it progresses rapidly to dementia and death. There may also be ataxia due to cerebellar degeneration. Prion disease can be inherited, infectious, or sporadic (of unknown cause). Inherited, or familial, prion disease is genetic. There are 20 known genetic mutations that cause prion disease. One of these is Creutzfeldt-Jakob disease. Infectious, or acquired, prion disease is transmitted by eating infected tissues or from medical procedures that use infected tissues. Sporadic prion disease may be due to one of the other two causes but without evidence of causation.

Thiamine deficiency (which can result from excessive alcohol intake, malnutrition, dialysis, severe morning sickness with vomiting during pregnancy, or prolonged administration of intravenous fluids without vitamins) can cause Wernicke-Korsakoff syndrome. About 10% of chronic alcoholics develop Wernicke-Korsakoff syndrome. Wernicke's syndrome is the early, or acute, stage of the disorder, and Korsakoff's amnesic syndrome is the chronic phase of the disorder. Wernicke's syndrome is characterized by ataxia, paralysis of certain eye muscles, and confusion. Hemorrhagic lesions of the walls of the cerebral aqueduct and the third and fourth ventricles may appear. At this stage of the disease, therapy with thiamine replacement can reverse most of the symptoms, although half of the patients who recover continue to have trouble walking. Left untreated, Wernicke's syndrome eventually leads to coma and death. In fact, 15 to 20% of patients who are hospitalized for Wernicke's syndrome do not survive.

As the disease progresses to the Korsakoff's stage, there is bilateral degeneration of the mammillary bodies, the septal nuclei, and the midline thalamic nuclei, which may include the dorsomedial nucleus and the anterior nucleus. Loss of hippocampal volume comparable to that seen in Alzheimer's disease may also play a role in the amnesic symptoms of the disease. Atrophy of other brain areas, including the cerebellum, occur as well. Severe impairments of antero- grade and sometimes retrograde memory occur with the Korsakoff's stage of the disease. Although recovery is much slower than with Wernicke's, treatment with thiamine will reverse some of the symptoms, but the memory loss is irreversible. Frequently, supervised living conditions are necessary for Korsakoff's patients.

PREVENTING BRAIN DISEASE
Scientists have found that the foods we eat, the amount of exer- cise we get, our level of mental activity, and even the air we breathe can affect the way our brains function. Free radicals, or molecules with unpaired electrons, are generated during normal cellular functions. **Antioxidant enzymes** in the body as well as **antioxidants** that we get in food normally do a good job in neutralizing free radicals before they steal electrons from DNA, cell membranes, and other cellular constituents and damage cells. However, if antioxidant defenses are low or free radicals are produced at a rate higher than these defenses can handle, disease can result. Free radicals are thought to be involved in aging processes and in a number of diseases, including Parkinson's and Alzheimer's disease. Eating lots of

dark or brightly colored fruits and vegetables and taking antioxidant supplements are a good way to protect the brain from free radicals. Other nutrients, including omega-3 fatty acids and the B vitamins, have also been shown to be important for brain health. Regular exercise not only increases cerebral blood flow but has been shown to increase neurogenesis. Mental activity increases synaptic connections and helps provide a reserve of these connections as the brain ages. Avoiding toxins in our water supply and in our environment also helps protect the brain. So how we take care of our brain can make a big difference in how well it functions and resists disease processes.

CONNECTIONS

Damage to the nervous system resulting from trauma or disease can have devastating effects. Loss of function due to damage to structures and pathways in the neuromuscular system can cripple a person. Autoimmune disease may attack receptors at neuromuscular junctions or the myelin of axons. Depending on where the damage takes place, degeneration of structures in the basal ganglia can produce inhibition or disinhibition of movement. Cerebellar damage can lead to problems with balance and gait. Epilepsy can cause twitches or convulsions of muscles, but it starts in the cerebral cortex and is caused by too many groups of neurons firing at the same time. Injury and disease of areas in the temporal, frontal, and parietal lobes can result in severe cognitive impairments. Injury to the brain due to stroke or trauma causes an enormous loss of life and a large number of disabling conditions each year. Dementias are usually progressive neurodegenerative diseases that affect the elderly. However, dementia can happen at an earlier age if the person experiences trauma, infection, autoimmune disease, or genetic problems. To date, scientists have not found cures for most nervous system impairments. Preventive measures in the form of improved diet, regular exercise, and safety precautions may be one way to prevent the disorders. Rehabilitative therapy for both physical and cognitive impairments may also help people who are affected. Continued research to understand the disease processes involved may yield an understanding of how to stop them. Again, those answers may be related to the normal physiological processes that maintain the health of the nervous system.

Glossary

Acetylcholine Neurotransmitter released by preganglionic autonomic neurons, motor neurons, postganglionic parasympathetic neurons, certain nuclei in the brainstem and basal forebrain, and interneurons in various brain structures.

Action potential Electrical impulse produced by depolarization of the neuronal membrane below its threshold. Carries the neural message down the axon.

Addiction Physical and psychological dependence on a drug that occurs after repeated use.

Adenohypophysis Anterior lobe of the pituitary gland. Synthesizes and releases hormones into the bloodstream.

Adrenal medulla The "core" of the adrenal gland. Releases norepinephrine and epinephrine when activated.

Ageusia A total loss of taste sensation.

Agonist Drug that mimics the action of a neurotransmitter at its receptor.

Alpha activity Electrical activity in the brain that creates regular brain waves at a rate of 8 to 12 cycles per second.

Alpha motor neuron Neuron in ventral gray matter of the spinal cord. Branches of its axon synapse on muscle fibers and transmit the nerve signal that causes them to contract.

Amnesia Loss of memory due to trauma or disease.

Amygdala Limbic system structure important in the regulation of emotion. Found in the medial temporal lobe.

Amygdalofugal pathway Input/output pathway for the basolateral and central nuclear divisions of the amygdala.

Analgesia Pain relief. One of the effects of opiates.

Anandamide One of the endogenous cannaboids found in the human brain. It binds to the same membrane receptor to which THC, the active ingredient in marijuana, binds.

Anomia Impairment in word finding, or the ability to recall the names of objects.

Anosmia A complete loss of the sense of smell.

Antagonist Drug, neurotransmitter, or other chemical that binds to a receptor and blocks the action of a neurotransmitter.

Anterior Toward the front.

Anterior commissure Fiber bundle that links the temporal cortices of the two hemispheres. A few anterior fibers link olfactory structures of the two hemispheres.

Anterograde amnesia Loss of the ability to remember new information.

Antidiuretic hormone See **Vasopressin**.

Antioxidants Chemicals that block the oxidation process by neutralizing free radicals. Natural antioxidants include Vitamin C, Vitamin E, Vitamin A, and bioflavonoids.

Antioxidant enzymes Enzymes that act as antioxidants. Include catalase, superoxide dismustase, and glutathione peroxidase.

Apraxia Problems performing learned skilled movement due to damage to the brain.

Aqueous humor Fluid which circulates in the space between the cornea and the lens.

2-Arachidonoyl An endogenous cannaboid. Binds to the cannaboid receptor, to which THC, the active ingredient of marijuana, also binds.

Arachnoid membrane The meningeal layer between the dura mater and the pia mater of the brain and spinal cord.

Arachnoid space Cerebrospinal fluid-filled space between the arachnoid membrane and the pia mater that provides cushioning for the brain and spinal cord.

Arachnoid trabeculae Spidery extensions between the arachnoid membrane and the pia mater.

Ascending reticular activating system (ARAS) Fiber pathway consisting of axons of cholinergic, dopaminergic, serotinergic, and noradrenergic brainstem nuclei. Functions to activate the cerebral cortex.

Association area Area of the cerebral cortex that associates and integrates sensory and/or motor information from primary areas.

Associative learning See **Classical conditioning**.

Glossary

Astrocyte Glial cell that provides nutritional and structural support for neurons.

Ataxia Uncoordinated movements associated with cerebellar damage or impairment of cerebellar function due to intoxication.

Auditory Pertaining to the sense of hearing.

Autoimmune disease Disease that results when the immune system attacks one of the body's own proteins as if it were a foreign protein.

Autonomic nervous system Division of the peripheral nervous system which controls the body's vital processes, such as heart rate, blood pressure, and rate of respiration.

Aversive stimuli Unpleasant stimuli, such as footshock or a bitter taste.

Axon Neuronal process (extension) that carries the neural signal away from the cell body toward another neuron.

Axon hillock The place where the cell body meets the axon. This is where an action potential is generated.

Basal ganglia A group of subcortical nuclei that lie beneath the lateral ventricles in the forebrain. Through their interconnections with the thalamus and cerebral cortex, they participate in the motivation, planning, and execution of movements.

Basic rest-activity cycle (BRAC) A proposed 90-minute cycle of rest and activity that occurs throughout the day and continues through the night as the sleep cycle.

Bed nucleus of the stria terminalis Thin C-shaped amygdalar nucleus that follows the stria terminalis as it follows the C-shape of the caudate nucleus. Its functions are similar to those of the central amygdalar nuclei.

Beta activity Electrical brain activity in which brain waves occur irregularly at a rate of 13 to 30 cycles per second.

Bipolar cell A bipolar neuron found in the middle, or bipolar layer of the retina. Transmits visual information from the photoreceptor cells to the ganglion cells.

Bipolar neuron A neuron that has two processes, a dendrite and an axon, that arise from opposite ends of the cell body. Most bipolar neurons are sensory neurons.

Blood-brain barrier Set of barriers that protects the brain by preventing most substances from entering the brain. Includes the tight junctions of the endothelial lining of the brain capillaries.

Brainstem Area of the brain extending from the diencephalon to the junction of the brain with the spinal cord. Includes the medulla, pons, and midbrain.

Broca's area Area in the left inferior (lower) frontal lobe that is involved in the production of speech. Also called the motor speech area.

Calcarine fissure (or sulcus) A deep infolding of the cerebral cortex from the pole (tip) of the occipital lobe to near the posterior end of the corpus callosum. The primary visual cortex covers the banks of this fissure.

Cardiac muscle Muscle found only in the heart. Responsible for the heart's contractions. Resembles striated muscle in appearance but is like smooth muscle in function.

Caudally Toward the tail end of the brain—away from the face.

Caudate nucleus One of the input nuclei of the basal ganglia. C-shaped structure which lies close to the lateral ventricle and actually forms the lateral wall and floor of the body of the lateral ventricle. Involved in cognition and the control of eye movements.

Cell theory Theory that states that the cell is the unit that makes up the structures of all living things.

Cerebellum Convoluted brain structure that lies dorsal to the brainstem and covers the fourth ventricle. Involved in motor skill learning, posture, and planning and coordinating movement. May be involved in higher cognitive processes as well.

Cerebral cortex Thin (1.5- to 4.5-mm) layer of gray matter covering the cerebral hemispheres. Contains primary sensory and primary motor areas, unimodal association areas for the individual senses, multimodal association areas for the integration of sensory information from different senses, and limbic areas.

Circadian pacemaker Suprachiasmatic nucleus. Controls the timing of the sleep/wake cycle and the daily rhythms of physiological functions.

Classical conditioning A type of learning in which a previously neutral stimulus becomes associated with (conditioned to) a stimulus that naturally produces a response. After conditioning, the previously neutral stimulus, now a conditioned stimulus, will elicit the same response as the neutral stimulus.

Glossary

Cochlea The snail-shaped part of the inner ear that contains the organ of Corti (the auditory sensory organ).

Cone Receptor cell in the retina that provides us with high-acuity vision and color vision. Cones are most active in bright light.

Consolidation Process by which information is stored in memory. Appears to involve synaptic changes.

Corticobulbar tract Fiber pathway that travels from the motor cortices (upper motor neurons) to the motor nuclei (lower motor neurons) of the cranial nerves and to associated interneurons in the reticular formation.

Corticospinal tract Fiber pathway that travels from the motor cortices (upper motor neurons) to the motor neurons (lower motor neurons) in the spinal cord. Divides into the lateral corticospinal tract and the ventral corticospinal tract just above the spinal cord at the pyramidal decussation in the medulla.

Contralateral On the opposite side of the body.

Cornea Transparent, dome-shaped structure that covers the front of the eye. Helps focus light rays on the retina.

Corpus callosum Commissure that connects the cerebral hemispheres. Largest of the brain's commissures.

Cribriform plate Part of the ethmoid bone that is directly above the nasal cavity. Contains tiny perforations through which the axons of the primary olfactory neurons can travel from the nasal cavity up to the olfactory bulb at the base of the brain.

Cytoplasm The thick, semiliquid substance that fills the interior of a cell.

Declarative memory Memory that is conscious and can be put into words. Includes episodic and semantic memory.

Deep sleep See **Slow-wave sleep**.

Delta activity Brain waves that occur at a rate of fewer than 3.5 cycles per minute.

Dementia Loss of cognitive functions due to disease of or damage to brain structures or pathways.

Dendrites Small branch-like extensions that come off a neuron, located at the opposite end of the cell from the axon.

Dendritic spine Small budlike extension of a dendrite on which the terminal button of another neuron synapses.

Dentate gyrus One of the structures that make up the hippocampal formation.

Desynchronized sleep See **REM sleep**.

Diffuse axonal injury (**DAI**) Injury to the brain resulting from the shearing of the axoplasm of nerve fibers during sudden acceleration/deceleration.

Dopamine Monoamine neurotransmitter of the catecholamine subclass.

Dorsal Toward the back side. In the brain, toward the top.

Dorsal root ganglion Cluster of cell bodies of bipolar neurons whose dendrites bring sensory information from the periphery and whose axons transmit that information to the central nervous system. Found in the dorsal root of each spinal nerve.

Dorsomedial thalamic nucleus Relay nucleus to the prefrontal association cortex for the amygdala, basal ganglia, hypothalamus, and olfactory system. Relays temperature, pain, and itch information to anterior cingulate gyrus. Also has direct reciprocal connections with the prefrontal cortex. Involved in emotions, learning and memory, and cognition.

Dura mater Tough outer meningeal layer of the brain and spinal cord. Lines the skull and vertebral canal.

Dysdiadochokinesia Inability to produce rapidly alternating movements.

Dysmetria Overshooting of a target while pointing.

Eardrum See **Tympanic membrane**.

Electroencephalogram (**EEG**) Paper or electronic record of electrical activity of the brain. Obtained using electrodes pasted to the scalp.

Electromyogram (**EMG**) Record of muscle activity recorded using electrodes attached to the chin.

Electro-oculogram (**EOG**) Record of eye movements recorded using electrodes attached near the eyes.

Glossary

Embolism Blockage of a blood vessel by a clot or other material carried in the bloodstream from another area of the body.

Encoding Process by which the brain acquires information to be stored in memory.

Endogenous opioids Neurotransmitters produced by the brain that bind to the same receptors that opiates such as heroin and morphine bind to. Examples of endogenous opioids are the enkephalins, dynorphins, and endorphins.

Enteric nervous system The neuronal network within the walls of the gastrointestinal tract that operates independently of the central nervous system. It is considered to be a division of the autonomic nervous system.

Entrainment Synchronization of a natural rhythm to an external stimulus, such as sunlight.

Ependymal cells A type of glial cell. Form the ependymal layer that lines the ventricles of the brain.

Episodic learning Learning that involves remembering events and the order in which they occur.

Episodic memory Memory of events and the order in which they occur.

Euphoria Intense (usually exaggerated) feeling of pleasure or well-being. Produced by most addictive drugs.

Explicit memory Declarative memory.

Extensor A muscle that causes a limb to straighten out.

Extracellular fluid The fluid that surrounds cells. Has a different concentration of ions from that of intracellular fluid, the fluid within cells.

Extrafusal muscle fibers Muscle fibers involved in skeletal movement.

Fasciculation Spasm of the fibers of a single motor unit.

Flexor A muscle that causes a limb to bend.

Foramen magnum Opening at the base of the skull around the junction of the medulla and the spinal cord.

Fornix Input/output pathway between the hippocampus and the septal nuclei and hypothalamus.

Fovea Small area at the center of the retina where light focuses. Only cones are found in this area, and vision is sharpest there.

Free nerve endings Nonencapsulated receptors distributed throughout the body. Found in the dermis, cornea, the gastrointestinal tract, joint capsules, ligaments, tendons, intramuscular connective tissue, the membranes covering bone and cartilage, and dental pulp. Detect pain and temperature (the majority), tickle sensations, pressure, crude touch, and possibly heat and cold.

Frontal lobe The part of each cerebral hemisphere that is found in front of the central sulcus and above the lateral sulcus.

Gamma-amino butyric acid (GABA) An amino acid transmitter in the brain that inhibits the firing of neurons.

Gamma motor neurons Small motor neurons that synapse on intra-fusal muscle fibers (stretch receptors) and adjust their sensitivity.

Ganglia Plural of ganglion.

Ganglion Group of neurons with similar functions found in the peripheral nervous system.

Ganglion cells Neurons found in the outermost layer of the retina. Their axons come together at the back of the eye to form the optic nerve.

Glia Cells of the central nervous system that are different from neurons. They provide a variety of supporting functions for neurons.

Globus pallidus One of the basal ganglia. Medial to the putamen (closer to the midline). Sends most of the outputs of the basal ganglia.

Golgi tendon organ An encapsulated receptor that detects muscle tension.

Gray matter Term used to describe areas of the brain and spinal cord where there are many neurons, which give the tissue a grayish color.

Hemispheric dominance Refers to the dominant role of one or the other cerebral hemisphere in a particular function.

Hemorrhagic Refers to the release of blood onto the surface of the brain (subdural hematoma), into the subarachnoid space, or into the brain tissue itself. The noun form is *hemorrhage*.

Glossary

Hippocampal commissure Fiber tract that interconnects the two hippocampi.

Hippocampal formation An older term that refers collectively to the three subdivisions of the hippocampus: the dentate gyrus, the hippocampus proper, and the subiculum.

Hippocampus Hippocampal formation.

Hippocampus proper The cornu ammonis (CA) subfields, CA1 through CA4, of the hippocampus. Information flows from orbital and other limbic cortices to the entorhinal cortex to the dentate gyrus to Field CA3 to Field CA1 to the subiculum to the entorhinal cortex and from there to widespread areas of the cerebral cortex.

Hyperpolarization Influx of negative ions that increase the membrane potential of a neuron and decrease the probability of an action potential.

Hypnagogic hallucination Dreamlike sights, sounds, or smells that occur just before falling asleep or just after awakening. Represents the occurrence of REM sleep accompanied by sleep paralysis during a waking state.

Hypogeusia A partial loss of the sense of taste.

Hyposmia A partial loss of the sense of smell.

Hypothalamic-pituito-adrenal (HPA) axis Refers to the series of hormones produced by the hypothalamus, pituitary, and adrenal gland during the stress response. CRH released by the hypothalamus stimulates the release of ACTH by the pituitary. ACTH then stimulates the release of cortisol from the adrenal cortex.

Hypothalamus Group of nuclei located beneath the thalamus in the diencephalon. Participates in control of multiple physiological and endocrine functions.

Immediate memory See **Short-term memory**.

Implicit memory Nondeclarative memory.

Instrumental conditioning A form of stimulus-response learning in which the learner associates a particular behavior with a reward or punishment. Behaviors that are rewarded increase; behaviors that are punished decrease.

Insula Area of the cerebral cortex found at the floor of the lateral fissure. Covered by the opercula of the frontal and temporal lobes.

Insular cortex The area of cortex at the floor of the lateral fissure. It can be seen by pulling back the opercula of the frontal and temporal lobes.

Intention tremor Shaking of a limb while the limb is in motion.

Intervertebral foramen Opening between two vertebrae through which a spinal nerve exits.

Intrafusal muscle fibers (or muscle spindles) Stretch receptors that contains fibers innervated by sensory and motor nerve endings. Attached at either end to extrafusal muscle fibers.

Inverse agonist Drug that binds to a receptor and has the opposite effect to that of the endogenous neurotransmitter.

Involuntary Automatic; not under conscious control.

Ionotropic receptor Receptor that has a central ion channel that is opened when the receptor is activated.

Ipsilateral On the same side of the body.

Iris The pigmented, muscular structure that controls the size of the pupil and gives the eyes their color.

Ischemic Caused by an interruption of the blood supply to an area. The noun form is *ischemia*.

Kinesthesia The sense that makes us aware of body movements. It comes from information received from receptors in the muscles, tendons, and joints.

Lateral geniculate nucleus Thalamic nucleus to which the optic tract projects.

Lateralization of function Hemispheric dominance.

Laterodorsal tegmental nuclei (LDT) Brainstem cholinergic nuclei that contribute fibers to the ascending reticular activating system (ARAS). They are active during REM sleep. These nuclei are located close to the junction of the pons and midbrain and next to the locus coeruleus.

Lens Transparent structure suspended behind the iris of the eye by muscles that contract and relax to change its shape for near and far vision. It helps focus light on the retina.

Glossary

Level of injury The most caudal vertebral segment below which there is a partial or complete absence of sensation and movement on both sides of the body.

Limbic system Interconnected diencephalic and telencephalic nuclei that are involved in emotions and memory and that regulate ingestive, aggressive, and reproductive behaviors. Structures include the hippocampal formation, amygdala, septal nuclei, hypothalamus, olfactory bulb, piriform olfactory cortex, and limbic cortex.

Locus The site in the brain where the electrical activity of a focal seizure originates.

Long-term memory Memory that is stored in the brain for a long time—as long as a lifetime. It has an enormous capacity and includes all the knowledge we have learned and all the events of our lives.

Lumbar cistern The space in the lower vertebral canal that is not occupied by the spinal cord but instead by spinal nerves that descend from the spinal cord to exit their appropriate intervertebral foramina. This area is where the needle used for a spinal tap is inserted.

Macula Area in the center of the retina where light focuses and where cones are the most heavily concentrated.

Medial geniculate nucleus Nucleus in the thalamus to which auditory information goes before being relayed to the primary auditory cortex.

Median forebrain bundle Fiber pathway through which axons of brainstem nuclei ascend and descend between brainstem nuclei and the cerebral cortex as well as subcortical nuclei. The fibers of the ascending reticular activating system (ARAS) travel up this pathway, and projections from the hypothalamus to the autonomic nervous system travel down this pathway.

Medulla Most posterior region of the hindbrain (brainstem). Transitions to the spinal cord at the foramen magnum.

Meissner's corpuscles Elongated encapsulated receptors located just beneath the epidermis in hairless skin, especially in the hands and feet. Numerous in the fingertips and, together with Merkel endings, responsible for fine tactile (touch) discrimination.

Meninges Protective membranes that surround and cover the brain and spinal cord.

Merkel ending Nonencapsulated touch receptor with a disk-shaped terminal that inserts into a Merkel cell in the basal layer of the epidermis of both hairless and hairy skin. Found in between hair follicles in hairy skin.

Metabotropic receptor Receptor whose activation results in the activation of a G protein, which either binds to an ion channel and causes it to open or activates a second messenger system that causes the ion channel to open.

Microglia Smallest glial cells. Engulf and destroy invading microbes and clean up debris after brain injury. Also secrete growth factors and cytokines.

Midbrain Most anterior region of the hindbrain (brainstem). Located just beneath the diencephalon.

Middle ear Air-filled region between the eardrum and the inner ear. A chain of three tiny bones (ossicles) carry vibrations from the eardrum to the oval window of the cochlea.

Monoamine oxidases Brain and liver enzymes that break down the monoamine neurotransmitters serotonin, dopamine, and norepinephrine.

Monoamines A group of neurotransmitters that includes serotonin, norepinephrine, and dopamine.

Motor learning The learning of skilled movements such as knitting, playing a musical instrument, or riding a bicycle. The movements become automatic over time.

Motor unit A motor neuron, its axons and dendrites, and the muscle fibers that it innervates.

Movement decomposition A condition that can result from damage to the cerebellum. Movements that are normally smooth decompose into a jerky series of discrete movements.

Multipolar neuron Neuron that has multiple dendritic trees and one long axon. Most neurons, including motor neurons and pyramidal cells, are of this type.

Muscle endplate The specialized area on the membrane of a muscle fiber on which the axon terminal of a motor neuron synapses. Nicotinic receptors are found inside the folds that increase the surface area of the synapse.

Muscle spindles Long, thin stretch receptors found scattered among muscle fibers. They detect changes in muscle length.

Glossary

Myelin Insulating covering formed by the concentric wrapping of oligodendrocyte or Schwann cell processes around an axon. Increases the conduction velocity of the axon.

Myofibrils Filaments (chains) of myosin or actin molecules.

Narcolepsy Sleep disorder in which a person is always sleepy during the daytime. Short episodes of REM sleep during waking hours are characteristic of this disorder.

Neural tube Embryonic precursor of nervous system. Cells lining the neural tube become neurons and glia, and the tube's cavity becomes the ventricular system and spinal canal.

Neurogenesis Production of new neurons from stem cells. Long thought to be absent in the adult brain of humans, but now known to occur in the hippocampus and in the lining of the lateral ventricles.

Neurohypophysis Posterior lobe of the pituitary.

Neuromuscular junction Synapse between alpha motor neuron and muscle fiber. Includes presynaptic motor terminal, synaptic cleft, and muscle endplate.

Neuron Nerve cell. Functional and structural unit of the nervous system.

Neuron theory The belief that the nervous system is made up of cells, in contrast to the reticular theory.

Neuropeptide Short peptide that functions as a neurotransmitter. Cleaved from larger precursor protein and transported from cell body to axon terminal.

Neurotransmitter Chemical messenger of the nervous system. Binds to a specific receptor and activates it.

Nociceptor Pain receptor. Consists of free nerve endings that receive and transmit information about harmful stimuli.

Node of Ranvier Gap between myelin wrappings of individual glial cells around the axon. Sodium ion channels concentrated here open to regenerate the axon potential as it travels from node to node down the axon in what is known as saltatory conduction.

Nondeclarative memory Stored information that is not available to conscious thought and is difficult to explain in words.

NonREM sleep The four stages of sleep that precede REM (rapid eye movement) sleep.

Norepinephrine A monamine neurotransmitter of the catecholamine subclass. It is produced and released by all sympathetic postganglionic neurons except those that innervate the sweat glands; by brainstem nuclei (of which the locus coeruleus is the most important); and by the adrenal medulla (as a hormone).

Nuclei Plural of *nucleus.*

Nucleus The control center of the cell. Contains the chromosomes.

Nucleus accumbens Structure in the ventral striatum that is formed by the fusion of the caudate nucleus and the putamen where they meet. It serves as an interface between the limbic system and the motor system and is also important in addiction and substance abuse.

Observational learning Learning by watching and mimicking the actions of others.

Occipital lobe Posterior lobe of the brain where the primary and association visual cortices are located.

Oculomotor loop Anatomical loop from the areas in the frontal and parietal lobe that control eye movements to the substantia nigra (one of the basal ganglia), then to the ventral anterior thalamic nucleus and back to the prefrontal and higher order visual cortices.

Olfactory receptors Proteins on the surface of primary olfactory neurons that detect gaseous molecules in the air.

Olfactory tract The nerve pathway from the olfactory bulb to the primary olfactory cortex.

Oligodendrocyte Glial cell that provides the myelin wrapping of axons in the central nervous system.

Optic chiasm Area directly above (dorsal to) the pituitary gland and directly below (ventral to) the hypothalamus where the nasal half of each optic nerve crosses to the contralateral side of the brain.

Optic radiation Nerve pathway from the lateral geniculate nucleus back through the temporal lobe to the ipsilateral primary visual cortex.

Orbitofrontal cortex Area of prefrontal cortex found at the base of (underneath) the brain. It gets its name from its location directly above the orbital bones of the eye sockets. It is the area of the frontal lobe that is most involved in emotions.

Glossary

Organelles Specialized intracellular structures found in the cytoplasm of a cell. They are each covered with a membrane and perform essential functions for the cell. Examples include the nucleus, mitochondria, the endoplasmic reticulum, and the ribosomes.

Organ of Corti The sensory organ of the inner ear. Consists of the tectorial membrane and all of the cells on its surface, including the hair cells.

Osmolarity A measure of the number of particles of a dissolved substance in liquid, such as plasma. Sodium, chloride, glucose, and urea are the substances that contribute the most to the osmolarity of plasma.

Osmoreceptors Receptors that detect changes in the osmolarity of the blood.

Ossicles The three tiny bones of the middle ear, called the malleus, incus, and stapes.

Outer ear Consists of the pinna, ear canal, and tympanic membrane.

Oxytocin Hypothalamic hormone that causes contraction of the uterus during labor and ejection of milk during nursing.

Pacinian corpuscles Encapsulated receptors that are widespread throughout the body in the subcutaneous tissue, especially in the hands and feet. Also found in the internal organs, joint capsules, and the membranes that line the internal cavity and support the organs. Particularly sensitive to vibration.

Paraplegia Injury of the spinal cord that results in a loss of sensation and movement that may occur anywhere from the middle of the chest down through the extremities.

Parasympathetic nervous system A division of the autonomic nervous system. Performs restorative and maintenance functions. Preganglionic neurons are found in the brainstem and the sacral spinal cord. Both its preganglionic and postganglionic neurons release the neurotransmitter acetylcholine.

Parietal lobe One of the four lobes of each cerebral hemisphere. It is bounded on the rear by the parieto-occipital sulcus, in the front by the central sulcus, and at the bottom by the lateral sulcus and an imaginary line that extends from the edge of the lateral sulcus and intersects at right angles with an imaginary line drawn from the parieto-occipital sulcus to the occipital notch.

Parieto-occipital sulcus Sulcus that forms the boundary between the parietal lobe and the occipital lobe.

Partial agonists Drugs that bind to receptors and produce less intense effects than a natural neurotransmitter would.

Pedunculopontine tegmental nuclei (PPT) Cholinergic nuclei found in the brainstem near the junction of the pons and the midbrain and close to the locus coeruleus. Contribute fibers to the ARAS, and are active during REM sleep.

Perception Interpretation by the brain of sensory stimuli that it receives from the sense organs.

Perceptual learning A type of learning that allows us to recognize and identify stimuli and to learn the relationships between stimuli.

Periaqueductal gray area Area of gray matter surrounding the cerebral aqueduct in the midbrain. Important in suppression of pain transmission and behavioral expression of emotions.

Peripheral nervous system All components of the nervous system that are not contained within the brain and spinal cord. Includes the sensory neurons, autonomic ganglia, and peripheral nerves.

Photopigment A pigment found in photoreceptor cells. When exposed to light, it undergoes chemical changes that cause ion channels in the membrane to open and generate an action potential.

Photoreceptor Neuron in the innermost retinal layer. Transduces light stimuli into neural signals.

Pia mater Innermost and most delicate of the three meningeal layers surrounding the brain and spinal cord.

Pinna The flap of skin and cartilage on the outside of the head that we usually think of as the "ear."

Pituitary gland Called the "master gland" because it secretes hormones that control the secretion of hormones by other endocrine glands.

Pons Brainstem region that lies between the midbrain and the medulla and is overlain dorsally by the cerebellum.

Posterior Toward the back.

Postganglionic fibers Axons of postganglionic neurons. Synapse on target organs or tissue. Release acetylcholine (parasympathetic) or norepinephrine (sympathetic) from their axon terminals.

Glossary

Prefrontal lobotomy Surgical procedure in which either the dorsal connections of the orbitofrontal cortex to the cingulate gyrus or its ventral connections to the diencephalon and temporal lobes are severed. Results in a loss of the ability to express emotions.

Preganglionic fibers Axons of autonomic preganglionic neurons. Their cell bodies are found in the intermediolateral gray matter of the spinal cord. They synapse on postganglionic neurons in the autonomic ganglia and release acetylcholine.

Primary olfactory neurons Neurons in the nasal cavity that have olfactory receptors. Their axons go up through tiny openings in the cribriform plate of the ethmoid bone to synapse on neurons in the olfactory bulbs, which are located at the base of the brain.

Primary visual cortex Area of the cerebral cortex to which raw visual data is transmitted to be processed. Located in the cortex inside the calcarine fissure.

Prion An abnormally folded protein that transmits disease when infected tissues are eaten. Resistant to inactivation by enzymes. Sometimes called a "slow virus."

Procedural memory Memories that result from motor learning and rules that are learned unconsciously.

Proprioception Position sense.

Pseudounipolar neuron A type of bipolar neuron that has a fused process that bifurcates a short distance from the cell body into an axon and a dendrite. The dorsal root ganglion cell is an example of a bipolar neuron.

Pupil The opening at the center of the iris of the eye.

Putamen A basal ganglia nucleus. Involved in the control of movements of the limbs and the trunk.

Quadriplegia See **Tetraplegia**.

Reflex Involuntary response to a stimulus.

Refractory period Period of a few milliseconds following an action potential in which at first another action potential cannot be generated (absolute refractory period) and then can be generated only with a much greater depolarization (relative refractory period). Results from inactivation of sodium channels.

Rehearsal Repetition of information in short-term memory. Increases the likelihood that it will be stored in long-term memory.

Relational learning Type of learning that involves learning relationships between multiple stimuli. Includes spatial learning, episodic learning, observational learning, and the more complex forms of perceptual learning.

REM sleep Period of sleep characterized by rapid eye movements, muscle atonia, vivid story-like dreams, and electrical activity similar to that seen during the waking state.

Renshaw cell Interneuron in the spinal cord that provides a negative feedback control for the alpha motor neuron.

Reticular formation Loose network of neurons and their processes that occupies most of the tegmentum (floor) of the brainstem. It receives afferents from all the senses, projects profusely upward and downward in the central nervous sytem, and is involved in virtually all activities of the central nervous system.

Reticular theory The belief that the nervous system is a network of cytoplasm with many nuclei but no individual cells.

Reticulospinal tract Fiber tract that descends from the reticular formation to the spinal cord and participates in the control of automatic movements such as walking and running, in the maintenance of muscle tone and posture, and in the control of sneezing, coughing, and respiration.

Retina Layer behind the vitreous humor and in front of the choroid. Consists of three layers of neurons that are interconnected by interneurons. The three layers of neurons are the inner photoreceptor layer, the middle bipolar layer, and the outer ganglion layer.

Retrieval The process by which information is accessed in the memory stores.

Retrograde amnesia Loss of memory for events that occurred before a trauma to the brain.

Rod Photoreceptor that is sensitive to light of low intensity and therefore helps us see in dim light. Does not contain color pigments, so it only allows us to see in tones of gray.

Rostrally Toward the head. In the brain, toward the face.

Rubrospinal tract Fiber tract that descends from the red nucleus down the contralateral brainstem and spinal cord. It is thought to be important in the control of the movements of arm and hand muscles but not the muscles of the fingers.

Glossary

Ruffini's corpuscles (or Ruffini's endings) Encapsulated receptors found in the dermis of hairy skin. Respond to stretch in the skin and to deep pressure. Capsules are cigar-shaped.

Satiety The feeling of fullness or satisfaction.

Schwann cell Glial cell that provides the myelin for peripheral nerves.

Sclera The tough white membrane that covers most of the eyeball (except the cornea).

Secondary visual cortex Area of cortex that is located on the outside of the calcarine fissure and surrounds the primary visual cortex, which is located inside the calcarine fissure. Processes the raw visual data that it receives from the primary visual cortex.

Second messenger Chemical that relays and amplifies the signal sent when a chemical molecule binds to a membrane receptor. Produced by the activation of an enzyme by a G protein that is activated by receptor activation.

Semantic memory Memory of factual knowledge as opposed to memory of events.

Sensation Receiving signals about the environment through the sense organs.

Sensory memory First stage of memory, which holds information for only milliseconds or seconds.

Serotonin A monamine neurotransmitter of the indoleamine subclass. Released from the raphe nuclei in the brainstem and in other places in the brain as well.

Short-term memory Second stage of memory, which can store 7 (plus or minus 2) items for a duration of seconds to minutes. (Also known as immediate memory or working memory.)

Skeletal muscles Voluntary muscles. Usually attached at each end to two different bones. When they contract, they cause the limbs and other structures to move.

Slow-wave sleep Stages 3 and 4 of nonREM sleep. Also known as deep sleep.

Smooth muscle Nonstriated muscle. Found in the muscles inside the eye, which control pupil size and the shape of the lens; in the sphincters of the urinary bladder and anus; in the walls of the blood vessels; in the walls of the digestive, urinary, and reproductive tracts; and around the hair follicles. Smooth muscle is under the control of the autonomic nervous system.

Somatic nervous system A division of the peripheral nervous system. Consists of the axons of the motor neurons and the sensory neurons and their axons.

Somatosensory Pertaining to the body senses: pain, touch, pressure, temperature, proprioreception, kinesthesia.

Spatial learning Learning about objects in the environment and their relative location to one another and to the learner.

Stimulus-response learning Occurs when a particular response to a stimulus is learned. Includes classical conditioning and instrumental conditioning.

Storage See **Consolidation**.

Stressors Stimuli that the brain perceives as a threat to the physical or emotional safety of the body or to its homeostasis (balance).

Stress response Physiological response to a stressor. Consists of the activation of the sympathetic nervous system, the noradrenergic system (locus coeruleus), and the HPA axis.

Stria terminalis Input/output pathway for the corticomedial nuclear group of the amygdala. Primary target is the hypothalamic ventro-medial nucleus.

Striations The darker stripes on skeletal muscles where myosin and actin filaments overlap.

Subiculum Structure of the hippocampal formation. Receives information from the hippocampus proper and projects it to the entorhinal cortex.

Substantia nigra A midbrain structure that is considered one of the basal ganglia. Projects to the striatum through a dopaminergic pathway. This pathway degenerates during Parkinson's disease.

Subthalamic nucleus One of the basal ganglia. Has reciprocal connections with the putamen. Damage to this nucleus causes hemiballism, or ballistic movements, of the contralateral limbs.

Sympathetic nervous system Division of the autonomic nervous system. Preganglionic neurons are found in the thoracic and lumbar intermediolateral area.

Synapse Refers to the combination of the synaptic cleft and the presynaptic and postsynaptic membranes.

Synaptic cleft The tiny space between two neurons across which the neurotransmitter released by the axon terminals of the presynaptic neuron travels to bind to receptors on the postsynaptic neuronal membrane.

Glossary

Synchronized sleep See **nonREM sleep**.

Synergistic Working together as a group.

Taste bud Onion-shaped taste organ that contains the taste receptor neurons. Most are found on or around the taste papillae on the surface of the tongue.

Tectospinal tract Fiber tract that arises in the superior colliculus and descends through the contralateral brainstem to the cervical spinal cord. It is involved in the control of trunk, shoulder, and neck movements, especially reflexive responses to auditory, visual, and possibly somatosensory stimuli. May be involved in the coordination of head and eye movements.

Temporal lobe One of the four lobes of each cerebral hemisphere. Its upper boundary is the lateral sulcus, and its posterior boundary is the occipital lobe.

Tetraplegia Loss of sensation and movement in all four limbs due to an injury in the cervical spinal cord.

Thalamus Group of nuclei located above the hypothalamus in the diencephalon. All sensory information except that of the olfactory sense relays here before being sent to the cortex.

Thermoreceptors Receptors in the hypothalamus that sense changes in the body temperature and send signals to the autonomic nervous system.

Transduction The process by which sensory receptors convert mechanical, chemical, or physical stimuli into nerve signals.

Tympanic membrane The eardrum. Membrane that covers the opening into the middle ear and vibrates in response to sound waves that enter the outer ear.

Unipolar neuron A neuron that has only one process, an axon, which has multiple terminals. Since there are no dendrites, the cell body receives all incoming information.

Vasoconstriction Narrowing or constriction of blood vessels. Activation of the sympathetic nervous system causes vasoconstriction. Other causes include disease and certain medications.

Vasopressin Antidiuretic hormone (ADH). Causes the kidney to reabsorb more water and decrease urine production. Also causes vasoconstriction, which produces an increase in blood pressure.

Ventral Referring to the front, or abdominal, side. In the brain, toward the lower side.

Ventricles Cavities within the brain that are filled with cerebrospinal fluid, which is secreted by the choroid plexus.

Ventricular system The continuous system of ventricles in the brain through which the cerebrospinal fluid circulates. It consists of the paired lateral ventricles in the cerebrum, the third ventricle in the diencephalon, the cerebral aqueduct in the midbrain, and the fourth ventricle between the cerebellum and the pons and medulla. Cerebrospinal fluid leaves the fourth ventricle through several small openings and bathes the brain and spinal cord.

Vermis Midline structure that connects the two hemispheres of the cerebellum.

Vertebral foramen The vertebral canal. The opening inside a vertebra in which a spinal cord segment lies.

Vestibule The middle cavity of the bony labyrinth of the inner ear. Lies between the semicircular canals and the cochlea. Contains the vestibular sacs: the saccule and the utricle.

Vestibulospinal tracts Two motor pathways from the vestibular nucleus to the spinal cord. The lateral vestibulospinal tract descends to all levels of the spinal cord and is important in the control of posture and balance. The medial vestibulospinal tract descends to the cervical and upper thoracic spinal cord and participates in the control of head position.

Vitreous humor The gel-like substance that fills the back of the eye and maintains the shape of the eyeball.

Voluntary Under conscious, deliberate control.

Wernicke's area Area located posterior to the primary auditory area of the left temporal lobe. Damage to this area results in impairment in language comprehension.

White matter Areas of the brain where fiber tracts predominate. These areas have a whitish appearance due to the myelin in the numerous axons.

Bibliography

Books and Journals

Abbott, N. J. "Astrocyte-endothelial Interactions and Blood-brain Barrier Permeability." *Journal of Anatomy* 200 (2002): 629–638.

Alva, G., and S. G. Potkin. "Alzheimer's Disease and Other Dementias." *Clinics in Geriatric Medicine* 19 (2003): 763–776.

American Psychiatric Association. *Task Force on Tardive Dyskinesia.* Washington, D.C.: American Psychiatric Association, 1992.

Berczi, I., and A. Szentivanyi. "The Immune-Neuroendocrine Circuitry." *Neuroimmune Biology Vol 3: The Immune-Neuroendocrine Circuitry: History and Progress*, eds. Istvan Berczi and Andor Szentivanyi. Boston: Elsevier, 2003, pp. 561–592.

Bloom, F., C. A. Nelson, and A. Lazerson. *Brain, Mind, and Behavior*, 3rd ed. New York: Worth Publishers, 2001.

Bouret, S. G., S. J Draper, and R. B. Simerly. "Formation of Projection Pathways from the Arcuate Nucleus of the Hypothalamus to Hypothalamic Regions Implicated in the Neural Control of Feeding Behavior in Mice." *Journal of Neuroscience* 24 (2004): 2797–2805.

Bowman, T. J. *Review of Sleep Medicine.* Boston: Butterworth Heinemann/ Elsevier Science, 2003.

Broadbent, N. J., R. E. Clark, S. Zola, and L. R. Squire. "The Medial Temporal Lobe and Memory." *Neuropsychology of Memory*, 3rd ed., eds. L. R. Squire and D. L. Schacter. New York: The Guilford Press, 2002, pp. 3–23.

Bruns, J., Jr., and W. A. Hauser. "The Epidemiology of Traumatic Brain Injury: A Review." *Epilepsia* 44 (Suppl. 10) (2003): 2–10.

Caplan, L. R. *Caplan's Stroke: A Clinical Approach*, 3rd ed. Boston: Butterworth-Heinemann, 2000.

Carlson, N. R. *Physiology of Behavior*, 6th ed. Boston: Allyn and Bacon, 1998.

Carlson, N. R., and W. Buskist. *Psychology: The Science of Behavior*, 5th ed. Boston: Allyn and Bacon, 1997.

Carper, J. *Your Miracle Brain.* New York: HarperCollins Publishers, 2000.

Castro, A. J., M. P. Merchut, E. J. Neafsey, and R. D. Wurster. *Neuroscience: An Outline Approach.* St. Louis, MO: Mosby Publishing, 2002.

Cheer, J. F., K. M. Wassum, M. L. A. V. Heien, P. E. M. Philips, and R. M. Wightman. "Cannaboids Enhance Subsecond Dopamine Release in the Nucleus Accumbens of Awake Rats." *The Journal of Neuroscience* 24 (2004): 4393–4400.

Chou, T. C., T. E. Scammell, J. J. Gooley, S. E. Gaus, C. B. Saper, and J. Lu. "Critical Role of Dorsomedial Hypothalamic Nucleus in a Wide Range of Behavioral Circadian Rhythms." *The Journal of Neuroscience* 23 (2003): 10691–10702.

Cooper, J. R., F. E. Bloom, and R. H. Roth. *The Biochemical Basis of Neuropharmacology*, 8th ed. New York: Oxford University Press, 2003.

D'Andrea, M. R. "Evidence Linking Neuronal Cell Death to Autoimmunity in Alzheimer's Disease." *Brain Research* 982 (2003): 19–30.

Doyon, J., and L. G. Ungerleider. "Functional Anatomy of Motor Skill Learning." *Neuropsychology of Memory*, 3rd ed., eds. L. R. Squire and D. L. Schacter. New York: The Guilford Press, 2002, pp. 225–238.

Duncan, J., and A. M. Owen. "Common Regions of the Human Frontal Lobe Recruited by Diverse Cognitive Demands." *Trends in Neurosciences* 23 (2000).

Ekdahl, C. T., J. H. Claasen, S. Bonde, Z. Kokaia, and O. Lindvall. "Inflammation Is Detrimental for Neurogenesis in Adult Brain." *Proceedings of the National Academy of Sciences, USA* 100 (2003): 13632–13637.

Finger, S. *Minds Behind the Brain: A History of the Pioneers and Their Discoveries.* Oxford: Oxford University Press, Inc, 2000.

Fitzgerald, M.J.T. *Neuroanatomy: Basic and Clinical*, 2nd ed. Philadelphia: Balliere Tindall, 1992.

FitzGerald, M.J.T., and J. Folan-Curran. *Clinical Neuroanatomy and Related Neuroscience*, 4th ed. New York: W. B. Saunders, 2002.

Florence, T. M. "Free Radicals in Parkinson's Disease." *Journal of Neurology* 249 Suppl 2 (2002):1–5.

Frey, L. C. "Epidemiology of Posttraumatic Epilepsy: A Critical Review." *Epilepsia* 44 (Suppl. 10) (2003): 11–17.

Gabry, K. E., G. Chrousos, and P. W. Gold. "The Hypothalamic-Pituitary-Adrenal (HPA) Axis: A Major Mediator of the Adaptive Responses to Stress." *Neuroimmune Biology Vol 3: The Immune-Neuroendocrine Circuitry: History and Progress*, eds. Istvan Berczi and Andor Szentivanyi. Boston: Elsevier, 2003.

Gazzaniga, M. D., R. B. Ivry, and G. R. Mangun. *Cognitive Neuroscience*, 2nd ed. New York: W. W. Norton and Company, 2002.

Gershberg, F. B., and A. P. Shimamura. "The Neuropsychology of Human Learning and Memory." *Neurobiology of Learning and Memory.* San Diego: Academic Press, 1998, pp. 33–359.

Gilman, S., and S. W. Newman. *Manter and Gatz's Essentials of Clinical Neuroanatomy and Neurophysiology*, 10th ed. Philadelphia: F. A. Davis Company, 1996.

Bibliography

Gleitman, H., A. J. Fridlund, and D. Reisberg. *Basic Psychology*, 5th ed. New York: W. W. Norton & Company, 2000.

Gluck, M. A., and C. E. Myers. "Psychobiological Models of Hippocampal Function in Learning and Memory." *Neurobiology of Learning and Memory*. San Diego: Academic Press, 1998, pp. 417–448.

Gray, P. *Psychology*, 3rd ed. New York: Worth Publishers, 1999.

Gronfier, C., and G. Brandenberger. "Ultradian Rhythms in Pituitary and Adrenal Hormones: Their Relations to Sleep." *Sleep Medicine Reviews* 2 (1998): 17–29.

Growdon, J. H., and N. R. Martin. *Blue Books of Practical Neurology: The Dementias*. Boston: Butterworth-Heinemann, 1998.

Hauser, W. A., and A. Pavone. "Introduction." *Epilepsia* 44 (Suppl. 10) (2003): 1.

Haines, D. E. *Fundamental Neuroscience*. Philadelphia: Churchill Livingstone, 2002.

Herd, J. A. "Cardiovascular Response to Stress." *Physiological Reviews* 71 (1991): 305–330.

Kennaway D. J., K. Lushington, D. Dawson, L. Lack, C. van den Heuvel, and N. Rogers, "Urinary 6-sulfatoxymelatonin Excretion and Aging: New Results and a Critical Review of the Literature." *Journal of Pineal Research* 27 (1999): 210–220.

Knowlton, B. J. "The Role of the Basal Ganglia in Learning and Memory." *Neuropsychology of Memory*, 3rd ed., eds. L. R. Squire and D. L. Schacter. New York: The Guilford Press, 2002, pp. 143–153.

Kolb, B., and I. Q. Whislaw. *An Introduction to Brain and Behavior*. New York: Worth Publishers, 2001.

Koutsilieri, E., Scheller, C., Grunblatt, E., Nara, K., Li, J., and Riederer, P. "The Role of Free Radicals in Disease." *Australian and New Zealand Journal of Ophthamology* 23 (1995): 3–7.

Kuchler, M., K. Fouad, O. Weinmann, M. E. Schwab, and O. Raineteau. "Red Nucleus Projections to Distinct Motor Neuron Pools in the Rat Spinal Cord." *Journal of Comparative Neurology* 448 (2002): 349–359.

Launer, L. J. "Dietary Anti-Oxidants and the Risk for Brain Disease: The Hypothesis and Epidemiologic Evidence." *Diet-Brain Connection: Impact on Memory, Mood, Aging and Disease*, ed. M. P. Mattson. Boston: Kluwer Academic Publishers, 2002.

Lavie, P. "Sleep-Wake as a Biological Rhythm." *Annual Review of Psychology* 52 (2001): 277–303.

Li, C., P. Chen, M. S. Smith. "Neuropeptide Y (NPY) Neurons in the Arcuate Nucleus (ARH) and Dorsomedial Nucleus (DMH), Areas Activated During Lactation, Project to the Paraventricular Nucleus of the Hypothalamus (PVH)." *Regulatory Peptides* 75–76 (1998): 93–100.

Mansvelder, H. D., M. D. Rover, D. S. McGehee, and A. B. Brussaard. "Cholinergic Modulation of Dopaminergic Reward Areas: Upstream and Downstream Targets of Nicotine Addiction." *European Journal of Pharmacology* 480 (2003): 117–123.

Martin, J. H. *Neuroanatomy: Text and Atlas*, 3rd ed. New York: McGraw-Hill Medical Publishing Division, 2003.

Martinez, J. L., Jr., E. J. Barea-Rodriguez, and B. E. Derrick. "Long-Term Potentiation, Long-Term Depression, and Learning." *Neurobiology of Learning and Memory*. San Diego: Academic Press, 1998, pp. 211–246.

Massion, J. "Red Nucleus: Past and Future." *Behavioral Brain Research* 28 (1988): 1–8.

McCurdy, M. L., D. I. Hansma, J. C. Houk, and A. R. Gibson. "Selective Projections From the Cat Red Nucleus to Digit Motor Neurons." *Journal of Comparative Neurology* 265 (1987): 367–379.

McGaugh, J. L. "The Amygdala Regulates Memory Consolidation." *Neuropsychology of Memory*, 3rd ed., eds. L. R. Squire and D. L. Schacter. New York: The Guilford Press, 2002, pp. 437–449.

Mecocci, P. "Oxidative Stress in Mild Cognitive Impairment and Alzheimer's Disease: A Continuum. *Journal of Alzheimer's Disease* 6 (2004): 159–63.

Meythaler, J. M., J. D. Peduzzi, E. Eleftheriou, and T. A. Novack. "Current Concepts: Diffuse Axonal Injury-Associated Traumatic Brain Injury." *Archives of Physical Medicine and Rehabilitation* 82 (2001): 1461–1471.

Mulder, A. B., M. G. Hodenpijl, and F. H. Lopes da Silva. "Electrophysiology of the Hippocampal and Amygaloid Projections to the Nucleus Accumbens of the Rat: Convergence, Segregation, and Interaction of Inputs." *Journal of Neuroscience* (1998): 5095–6102.

Nance, D. M., and B. J. MacNeil. "Immunoregulation by Innervation. The Immune-Neuroendocrine Circuitry." *Neuroimmune Biology Vol 3: The Immune-Neuroendocrine Circuitry: History and Progress*, eds. Istvan Berczi and Andor Szentivanyi. Boston: Elsevier, 2003.

Nathan, P. W., and M. C. Smith. "The Rubrospinal and Central Tegmental Tracts in Man." *Brain* 105 (Pt 2) (1982): 223–269.

Bibliography

Nathans, J., T. P. Piantanida, R. L. Eddy, T. B. Shows, and D. S. Hogness. "Molecular Genetics of Inherited Variation in Human Color Vision." *Science* 232 (1986): 203–210.

Nestler, E. J. "Common Molecular and Cellular Substrates of Addiction and Memory." *Neurobiology of Learning and Memory* 78 (2002): 637–647.

———. "Total Recall—The Memory of Addiction." *Science* 292 (2001): 2266–2267.

Nolte, J. *The Human Brain: An Introduction to Its Functional Anatomy*, 5th ed. St. Louis: Mosby Publishing, 2002.

Oades, R. D., and G. M. Halliday. "Ventral Tegmental (A10) System: Neurobiology. 1. Anatomy and Connectivity." Brain Research Reviews (1987): 117–165.

Palkovits, M., and M. Fodor. "Distribution of Neuropeptides in the Human Lower Brainstem (Pons and Medulla Oblongata)." *Neurotransmitters in the Human Brain*, eds. D. J. Tracey et al. New York: Plenum Press, 1995, pp. 101–113.

Pavone, P., R. Bianchini, E. Parano, G. Incorpora, R. Rizzo, L. Mazzone, and R. R. Trifiletti. "Anti-brain Antibodies in PANDAS Versus Uncomplicated Streptococcal Infection." *Pediatric Neurology* 30 (2004): 107–110.

Roitt, I., J. Brostoff, and D. Male. *Immunology*, 5th ed. Philadelphia: Mosby, 1998.

Rolls, E. T. "Memory Systems in the Brain." *Annual Review of Psychology* 51. (2000) 599–630.

Russo, E. "Controversy Surrounds Memory Mechanism." *The Scientist* 13 (1999): 1.

Shneerson, J. M. *Handbook of Sleep Medicine*. Malden, MA: Blackwell Science Ltd., 2000.

Snell, R. S. *Clinical Neuroanatomy: An Illustrated Review with Questions and Explanations*, 3rd ed. Philadelphia: Lippincott, Williams & Wilkins, 2001.

Song, C., and B. E. Leonard. *Fundamentals of Psychoneuroimmunology*. New York: John Wiley & Sons, 2000.

Sullivan, E. V., and L. Marsh. "Hippocampal Volume Deficits in Alcoholic Korsakoff's Syndrome." *Neurology* 61 (2003): 1716–1719.

Swaab, D. F. *Handbook of Clinical Neurology Vol. 80* (3rd Series, Vol. 2). *The Human Hypothalamus: Basic and Clinical Aspects, Part I: Nuclei of the Human Hypothalamus*. Boston: Elsevier, 2004.

———. *Handbook of Clinical Neurology*, Vol. 80 (3rd Series, Vol. 2) *The Human Hypothalamus: Basic and Clinical Aspects, Part II: Neuropathology of the Human Hypothalamus and Adjacent Structures.* Boston: Elsevier, 2004.

Thompson, R. H., N. S. Canteras, and L. W. Swanson. "Organization of Projections From the Dorsomedial Nucleus of the Hypothalamus: A PHA-L Study in the Rat." *Journal of Comparative Neurology* 376 (1996): 143–173.

Usuda, I., K. Tanaka, and T. Chiba. "Efferent Projections of the Nucleus Accumbens in the Rat with Special Reference to Subdivision of the Nucleus: Biotinylated Dextran Amine Study." *Brain Research* (1998): 73–93.

Waxman, S. G. *Clinical Neuroanatomy.* New York: Lange Medical Books, 2003.

White, N. M. "Addictive Drugs as Reinforcers: Multiple Partial Actions on Memory Systems." *Addiction* 91 (1996): 921–949.

Wise, R. A. "Drug-activation of Brain Reward Pathways." *Drug and Alcohol Dependence* 51 (1998):13–22.

Wolf, M. E. "Addiction: Making the Connection Between Behavioral Changes and Neuronal Plasticity in Specific Pathways." *Molecular Interventions* 2 (2002): 146–157.

Websites

The Anatomy of a Head Injury:
http://www.ahs.uwaterloo.ca/~cahr/headfall.html

Autoimmune Disease Research Center at the Johns Hopkins Medical Institution:
http://autoimmune.pathology.jhmi.edu/

Autoimmune Disease Research Foundation:
www.cureautoimmunity.org/Science%20release.htm

B. F. Skinner:
http://www.ship.edu/~cgboeree/skinner.html

The Brain & the Actions of Cocaine, Opiates, and Marijuana:
http://www.udel.edu/skeen/BB/Hpages/Reward%20&%20Addiction2/actions.html

Brief Biography of B. F. Skinner:
http://www.bfskinner.org/bio.asp

Can Christopher Reeve Get Off the Ventilator?:
http://www.pulmonaryreviews.com/jan03/pr_jan03_superman.html

Bibliography

CDC: Fetal Alcohol Syndrome:
http://www.cdc.gov/ncbddd/fas/default.htm

Cerebral Ventricular System and Cerebrospinal Fluid
http://www.umanitoba.ca/faculties/medicine/anatomy/cv.htm

Chemical Warfare Primer:
http://www.mnpoison.org/index.asp?pageID=146

Chemical Weapons: Nerve Agents:
http://faculty.washington.edu/chudler/weap.html

Cocaine Addiction Linked to a Glutamate Receptor:
http://www.biomedcentral.com/news/20010829/04/

Cognitive Rehabilitation: What Is It?:
http://cogrehab.home.pipeline.com/cogrehab.htm

Conditioned Emotional Reactions:
http://psychclassics.yorku.ca/Watson/emotion.htm

The Ear:
http://medic.med.uth.tmc.edu/Lecture/Main/ear.htm

Embryological Development of the Human Brain:
www.newhorizons.org/neuro/scheibel.htm

The Enteric Nervous System:
*http://arbl.cvmbs.colostate.edu/hbooks/pathphys/digestion/basics/
gi_nervous.html*

The Enteric Nervous System: A Second Brain:
http://www.hosppract.com/issues/1999/07/gershon.htm

The Eye:
http://medocs.ucdavis.edu/cha/402/lectsyl/98/eye.HTM

Feuerstein's Instrumental Enrichment Program: Basic Theory:
http://www.icelp.org/asp/Basic_Theory.shtm

Free Radicals and Human Disease:
http://www.drproctor.com/crcpap2.htm

From Neurobiology to Treatment: Progress Against Addiction:
*http://www.nature.com/cgi-taf/DynaPage.taf?file=/neuro/journal/v5/
n11s/full/nn945.htmlUT*

Gulf War Syndrome Defined—Evidence and Conclusions:
http://members.cox.net/linarison/gws.html

Gulf War Syndrome Research Reveals Present Danger:
http://www.newscientist.com/news/news.jsp?id=ns99993546

How CAT Scans Work:
http://science.howstuffworks.com/cat-scan.htm

How MRI Works:
http://electronics.howstuffworks.com/mri.htm

The Internet Stroke Center: About Stroke:
http://www.strokecenter.org/pat/about.htm

Is Mercury Toxicity an Autoimmune Disorder?:
http://www.thorne.com/townsend/oct/mercury.html

Korsakoff's Syndrome:
http://www.chclibrary.org/micromed/00054130.html

The Mayo Clinic: Spinal Cord Injury:
http://www.mayoclinic.com/invoke.cfm?id=DS00460

Medline Plus: Taste—Impaired:
http://www.nlm.nih.gov/medlineplus/ency/article/003050.htm

Medline Plus: Spinal Cord Injuries:
http://www.nlm.nih.gov/medlineplus/spinalcordinjuries.html

Melatonin: A Review:
http://www.priory.com/mel.htm

Melatonin Information and References:
http://www.aeiveos.com/diet/melatonin/

Modulation of Prefrontal Cortex (PFC) and Fusiform Face Area (FFA) Responses to Increased Working Memory Demand for Faces:
http://www.uchsc.edu/sm/mstp/aspen99/html/oralhtml/oral_Druzgal_J.html

Monell Chemical Senses:
http://www.monell.org/

MS Information Sourcebook:
http://www.nationalmssociety.org/Sourcebook.asp

Nathaniel Kleitman (1895–1999):
http://www.uchospitals.edu/news/1999/19990816-kleitman.php

Neuroanatomy and Physiology of the "Brain Reward System" in Substance Abuse:
http://ibgwww.colorado.edu/cadd/a_drug/essays/essay4.htm

Neurotransmitter Systems I:
http://artsci-ccwin.concordia.ca/psychology/psyc358/Lectures/transmit1.htm

NINDS: Neurological Disorders and Disease Index:
http://www.ninds.nih.gov/health_and_medical/disorder_index.htm

Oral Cavity and Teeth:
http://medic.med.uth.tmc.edu/Lecture/Main/tool2.htm

Bibliography

Overview of Hypothalamic and Pituitary Hormones:
*http://arbl.cvmbs.colostate.edu/hbooks/pathphys/endocrine/hypopit/
overview.html*

Parasomnias (Sleep Walking, Sleep Talking, and Sleep Eating):
http://www.sleepdoctor.com/sw_st.htm

Pathophysiology of AD: Free Radicals:
*http://www.alzheimersdisease.com/hcp/about/patho/hcp_free_radicals
.jsp?checked=y*

Patient H. M.:
http://www.psy.ohio-state.edu/psy312/deniz-hm.html

The Phineas Gage Information Page:
http://www.deakin.edu.au/hbs/GAGEPAGE

The Physiology of Taste:
*http://www.sff.net/people/mberry/taste.htmPrion Diseases and the
BSE Crisis*

Pick's Disease Pathology: Pick Bodies:
http://www.binderlab.northwestern.edu/pickbodies.html

The Pleasure Centres Affected by Drugs
*http://www.thebrain.mcgill.ca/flash/i/i_03/i_03_cr/i_03_cr_par/i_03
_cr_par.html*

Prion Diseases and the BSE Crisis:
http://www.sciencemag.org/feature/data/prusiner/245.shl

The Prion Theory:
*http://www.portfolio.mvm.ed.ac.uk/studentwebs/session2/group4/
evidence.htm*

The Role of Sleep in Memory
http://www.memory-key.com/NatureofMemory/sleep_news.htm

Second Messengers:
*http://users.rcn.com/jkimball.ma.ultranet/BiologyPages/S/Second_
messengers.html*

Simple Anatomy of the Retina:
http://webvision.med.utah.edu/sretina.html

Sleep and Language:
http://thalamus.wustl.edu/course/sleep.html

Sleep Deprivation:
*http://www.macalester.edu/~psych/whathap/UBNRP/sleep_deprivation/
titlepage.html*

Smell and Taste Disorders:
http://www.entnet.org/healthinfo/topics/smell_taste.cfm

Southwestern's Eric J. Nestler on the Molecular Biology of Addiction:
   http://www.sciencewatch.com/nov-dec2001/sw_nov-dec2001_page3.htm

Skeletal Development in Human: A Model for the Study of Developmental Genes:
   http://www.infobiogen.fr/services/chromcancer/IntroItems/GenDevelLongEngl.html

SPINALCORD: Spinal Cord Injury Information Network:
   http://www.spinalcord.uab.edu

The Stages of Sleep:
   http://www.silentpartners.org/sleep/sinfo/s101/physio4.htm

The Strange Tale of Phineas Gage:
   http://www.brainconnection.com/topics/?main=fa/phineas-gage

Stress:
   http://www.neuroanatomy.wisc.edu/coursebook/neuro4(2).pdf

Substances of Abuse and Addiction:
   http://abdellab.sunderland.ac.uk/lectures/addiction/opiates1.html

Tardive Dyskinesia/Tardive Dystonia:
   http://www.breggin.com/tardivedysk.html

Taste—A Brief Tutorial by Tim Jacob:
   http://www.cf.ac.uk/biosi/staff/jacob/teaching/sensory/taste.html

That's Tasty:
   http://faculty.washington.edu/chudler/tasty.html

Toxicity, Organophosphates:
   http://www.emedicine.com/ped/topic1660.htm

Transport Across Cell Membranes:
   http://users.rcn.com/jkimball.ma.ultranet/BiologyPages/D/Diffusion.html

Traumatic Brain Injury: Definition, Epidemiology, Pathophysiology:
   http://www.emedicine.com/pmr/topic212.htm

What Is the Function of the Various Brain Waves?:
   http://brain.web-us.com/brainwavesfunction.htm

Further Reading

Books and Journals

Alexander, R. M. *The Human Machine.* New York: Columbia University Express, 1992.

Alzheimer's Disease: Unraveling the Mystery. National Institute on Aging, NIH Publication No. 02-3782, October 2002.

Baddeley, A. D. *Your Memory: A User's Guide.* London: Prion, 1993.

Blaylock, R. L. *Excitotoxins: The Taste That Kills.* Santa Fe: Health Press, 1997.

Bowman, J. P., and F. D. Giddings. *Strokes: An Illustrated Guide to Brain Structure, Blood Supply, and Clinical Signs.* Upper Saddle River, NJ: Prentice Hall, 2003.

The Brain Atlas. Bethesda, MD: Fitzgerald Science Press, Inc., 1998.

Hoffer, A., and M. Walker. *Smart Nutrients: Prevent and Treat Alzheimer's, Enhance Brain Function.* Garden City, NY: Morton Walker, 1994.

Matthews, G. G. *Introduction to Neuroscience (11th Hour).* Malden, MA: Blackwell Science, Inc., 2000.

Osborn, C. L. *Over My Head : A Doctor's Own Story of Head Injury From the Inside Looking Out.* Andrews McMeel Publishers, 1998.

Philpott, W. P., and D. K. Kalita. *Brain Allergies: The Psychonutrient and Magnetic Connections.* Los Angeles: Keats Publications, 2000.

Rolls, E. T. "Memory Systems in the Brain." *Annual Review of Psychology* 51 (2000): 599–630.

Springer, S. P., and G. Deutsch. *Left Brain, Right Brain: Perspectives from Cognitive Neuroscience,* 5th ed. New York: W. H. Freeman and Company, 1998.

Whalley, L. *The Aging Brain.* New York: Columbia University Press, 2001.

Websites

Animated Tutorials: Neurobiology/Biopsychology:
http://www.sumanasinc.com/webcontent/anisamples/neurobiology/neurobiology.html

The Brain:
http://www.enchantedlearning.com/subjects/anatomy/brain/index.shtml

Brain Connection:
http://www.brainconnection.com/

Brain Science (Author's Website):
http://groups.msn.com/BrainScience

BrainSource.com:
http://www.brainsource.com/

Brain Work:
http://www.dana.org/books/press/brainwork/

A Brief Introduction to the Brain:
http://ifcsun1.ifisiol.unam.mx/Brain/segunda.htm

Dana.org:
http://www.dana.org

Explore the Brain and Spinal Cord:
http://faculty.washington.edu/chudler/introb.html

How Your Brain Works:
http://science.howstuffworks.com/brain.htm

Milestones in Neuroscience Research:
http://www.univ.trieste.it/~brain/NeuroBiol/Neuroscienze%20per
%20tutti/hist.html

NeuralLinks Plus:
http://spot.colorado.edu/~dubin/bookmarks/index.html

Neuroscience:
http://cte.rockhurst.edu/neuroscience/page/outline.shtml

Neuroscience: A Journey Through the Brain:
http://ntsrv2000.educ.ualberta.ca/nethowto/examples/edit435/
M_davies/Neuroscience%20Web/index.htm#

Neuroscience Education:
http://faculty.washington.edu/chudler/ehceduc.html

Neuroscience Tutorial:
http://thalamus.wustl.edu/course

Neuroscience Links:
http://www.iespana.es/neurociencias/links.htm

Conversion Chart

Unit (metric)		Metric to English		English to Metric	
LENGTH					
Kilometer	km	1 km	0.62 mile (mi)	1 mile (mi)	1.609 km
Meter	m	1 m	3.28 feet (ft)	1 foot (ft)	0.305 m
Centimeter	cm	1 cm	0.394 inches (in)	1 inch (in)	2.54 cm
Millimeter	mm	1 mm	0.039 inches (in)	1 inch (in)	25.4 mm
Micrometer	μm				
WEIGHT (MASS)					
Kilogram	kg	1 kg	2.2 pounds (lbs)	1 pound (lbs)	0.454 kg
Gram	g	1 g	0.035 ounces (oz)	1 ounce (oz)	28.35 g
Milligram	mg				
Microgram	μg				
VOLUME					
Liter	L	1 L	1.06 quarts	1 gallon (gal)	3.785 L
				1 quart (qt)	0.94 L
				1 pint (pt)	0.47 L
Milliliter	mL or cc	1 mL	0.034 fluid ounce (fl oz)	1 fluid ounce (fl oz)	29.57 mL
Microliter	μL				
TEMPERATURE					
$°C = 5/9 \ (°F - 32)$		$°F = 9/5 \ (°C + 32)$			

Index

Index

Index

Index

Index

Picture Credits

About the Author

Dr. F. Fay Evans-Martin has a dual background in the areas of pharmacology and biopsychology. She holds degrees in biology (B.S.), pharmacology (M.S.), and psychology (Ph.D.) Her postdoctoral research was conducted in spinal cord injury at the University of Alabama at Birmingham and in nicotine self-administration at the University of Pittsburgh. Primary research interests are in learning and memory and neuroprotection. Dr. Evans-Martin is the mother of two sons.